KIDNEY DISEAS

FOR SENIORS ON STAGE 3

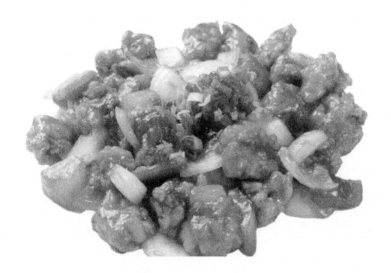

Comprehensive Guide for Managing Stage 3 CKD Through Delicious Low Sodium, Low Phosphorus and Low Potassium Kidney-friendly Recipes.

MICHELLE GREEN

FREE EMAIL CONSULTATION

Dear Reader,

Thank you for purchasing my book. As a token of my appreciation, I would like to offer you a free email consultation to help you clarify any concern in this book to your specific situation.

I understand that sometimes reading a book can raise questions or concerns, and you may be unsure about how to proceed. That's why I am here to help.

To take advantage of this offer, simply send me an email at michellediets101@gmail.com with the subject line "Book Consultation" and provide a brief description of the issue you would like to discuss. I will do my best to respond within 24 hours with actionable advice that will help you achieve your goals.

Please note that this offer is only available to readers who have purchased a copy of my book.

Thank you again for choosing to purchase my book, and I look forward to hearing from you soon.

MY OTHER BOOKS

I have other books that you could find helpful. Kindly scan the code below to gain access.

OR

https://www.amazon.com/author/michgreen

CONTENTS

INTRODUCTION

I'm so glad you picked up this cookbook. If you're reading this, chances are, you or someone you love is navigating the ups and downs of kidney disease. First off, I want to say—you're not alone. As a renal dietitian, I've walked alongside many people facing the same challenges. And while it's not an easy path, I've seen time and time again how food can be a powerful tool for both healing and connection. I'd like to start by sharing two stories that are close to my heart.

A few years back, I got a call from my friend Alicia. Her father, Charles, had just been diagnosed with Stage 3 kidney disease. Now, Charles wasn't just your average guy—he was full of life, loved his steaks, his Friday night pizzas, and pretty much anything hearty. Alicia was shaken. "Dad's always been so strong," she said, trying to keep it together. "Now it feels like he's slipping away, and we don't know how to help."

Shortly after that, Grace, a young woman who had just gotten engaged to my cousin, called me. Her Aunt Jane, the heart and soul of their family, was going through the same thing. Jane was the kind of person who made every family gathering feel special, mostly thanks to her legendary apple pies and those warm Sunday brunches. "I just can't imagine our family without her pies, her laugh, her presence," Grace told me, clearly heartbroken.

When I sat down with Charles and Jane, I could see it wasn't just the diagnosis weighing them down. They were both afraid that their love of food and the joy it brought to their families was over. Charles joked, "So, I guess I'm stuck with bland food forever, huh?" while Jane admitted she was terrified of losing the one thing that had always brought her loved ones together—her cooking.

But here's the thing—kidney-friendly eating doesn't have to be boring or restrictive. Together, we explored new ways of cooking, and soon, both Charles and Jane started to see food differently. Charles took to experimenting with herbs and spices, and before long, he was whipping up dishes that not only supported his health but brought back his love for cooking. I remember him saying, "I can't believe this is good for me—it's actually delicious!"

Jane, who was initially hesitant, found herself embracing the challenge, too. She started tweaking her recipes, discovering that with a few small changes, she could still make her famous dishes. Her kitchen was soon filled with the laughter and warmth it always had as her family gathered to enjoy her meals once again. "This isn't just about my health," she said to me one day, smiling. "It's about keeping my family close and celebrating life together."

Their stories are just a couple of examples of what I've seen countless times. A kidney disease diagnosis can feel overwhelming, but it's not the end. In fact, it can be the beginning of something new—a different way to experience food and family.

This book isn't just about recipes. It's about hope, resilience, and reclaiming the joy of cooking and eating, even with kidney disease. It's for anyone who wants to take back control, who refuses to let a diagnosis define them or take away life's simple pleasures. To Charles, Jane, and everyone else who's navigating this journey— you are stronger than you know. This cookbook is a tribute to that strength, and I hope it helps you see that your story is far from over. In fact, it's just getting started.

Are you ready to discover new ways to enjoy food and life again? Let's dive in together.

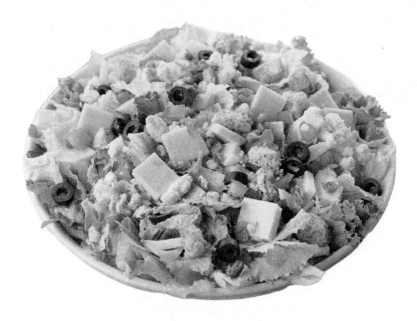

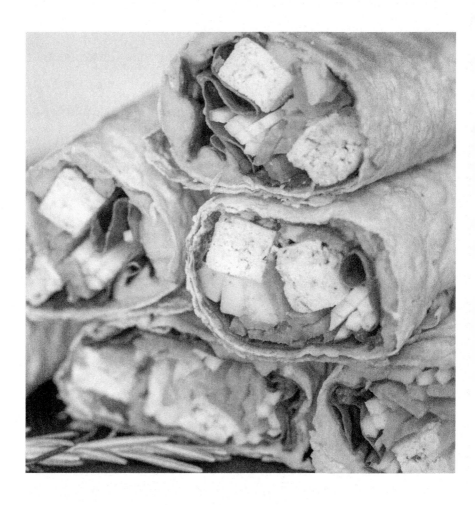

CHAPTER 1

UNDERSTANDING STAGE 3 KIDNEY DISEASE & YOUR DIET

Did you know that millions of seniors have kidney disease? Chronic kidney disease affects around 37% of seniors over the age of 65. Changes in our kidneys are natural as we age, and for many, this might progress to Stage 3 renal disease. Navigating life with stage 3 kidney disease may feel scary at first, but understanding the condition and how what you eat affects your health may make a big difference.

This chapter explains what Stage 3 entails, how it affects your health, and the crucial role your diet fulfils in preserving your health and strength.

Your Kidney And Their Vital Role

The kidneys are absolutely wonderful organs. These two bean-shaped workhorses, positioned near your spine, carry out a variety of functions that are critical to your overall health. Think of them as the body's internal cleaning team and master balancers. They filter your blood, eliminate waste products, regulate fluids to prevent swelling, assist in control of your blood pressure, and even help keep your bones healthy by controlling calcium and phosphate levels.

What Is Stage 3 Kidney Disease?

As we age, our bodies naturally change, and our kidneys are no exception. Stage 3 chronic kidney disease (CKD) indicates that your kidneys are moderately damaged. They're still filtering your blood, but they're not as effective as they previously were. The stage of CKD is determined by doctors using a value known as eGFR (estimated glomerular filtration rate), which measures how efficiently your kidneys filter waste. This stage is divided into two:

Stage 3A: eGFR ranges between 45 and 59 ml/min/1.73 m².

Stage 3B: the eGFR declines between 30 and 44 ml/min/1.73 m².

It's vital to have an understanding that Stage 3 kidney disease does not indicate your kidneys are no longer functional. Consider it an older automobile that still works well but requires further maintenance to keep it going strong. With proper care and lifestyle adjustments, persons with Stage 3 CKD can lead full and active lives.

Causes and Risk Factors

Several factors can lead to the development of Stage 3 kidney disease, which is frequently caused by other health conditions, including:

High Blood Pressure: Uncontrolled high blood pressure over time strains the tiny blood vessels in the kidneys.

Diabetes: High blood sugar levels can harm the delicate filtering units of the kidneys.

Other conditions: other risk factors include heart disease, autoimmune illnesses, and a family history of renal issues.

Symptoms

Kidney disease generally presents with no evident symptoms in its early stages, including Stage 3. As the condition advances, you may notice the following:

- Swelling in the feet, ankles, or hands
- Changes in urination
- Fatigue and difficulty concentrating
- Itchy or dry skin
- Loss of appetite
- Muscle cramps due to fluid and electrolyte imbalances.

The Power of Food and Why You Should Make Dietary Changes Now

When you have Stage 3 renal disease, your dietary choices have a big influence on your overall health. Certain foods might put additional strain on your kidneys, but others provide the necessary support. The good news is that a kidney-friendly diet does not have to be restricted or bland. With a few tweaks, you may eat nutritious and enjoyable meals that benefit your kidney health.

Dietary adjustments are designed to protect your kidneys, improve your general health, and decrease the course of kidney disease. Here's why it matters.

Prevents Further Damage: Eating kidney-friendly meals reduces the strain on your kidneys and helps keep them functioning for as long as possible.

Heart Health Benefits: Kidney health and heart health are inextricably linked. A kidney-friendly diet is deemed to be good for the heart, too.

Improves Energy Levels: Less waste buildup in the body from the kidneys can help you feel less fatigued and boost your energy levels.

Manage Other Conditions: A kidney-friendly diet aligns with healthy eating for blood pressure control, diabetes, and other common health issues among seniors.

Understanding Stage 3 kidney disease and the importance of food is the first step. In the next chapters, we will put this knowledge into action! You'll learn about tasty, kidney-friendly foods, meal-planning strategies, and ways to make these adjustments less stressful. Remember, it's all about safeguarding your health, feeling your best, and taking control of your well-being through the foods you consume.

CHAPTER 2

DIETARY GUIDELINES FOR STAGE 3 KIDNEY HEALTH

Managing Stage 3 renal disease requires paying particular attention to certain components in your diet. While this may appear challenging at first, understanding how these essential nutrients affect your health is really profound. In this chapter, we'll look at the dietary rules that will help preserve your kidneys, support your heart, and keep you feeling great. We'll cover everything from salt and potassium to protein and fluids, so you can confidently prepare nutritious and tasty meals.

How To Manage Your Sodium Intake

For individuals with Stage 3 kidney disease, salt is more than just a flavor enhancer. It's a key player in managing your overall health. Imagine sodium as a magnet in your body, absorbing and retaining water. The higher your salt intake, the more fluid your system tends to hold onto. This delicate balance can significantly impact your blood pressure and fluid levels, making sodium management a crucial aspect of kidney care.

Why Is This An Issue For Your Kidneys?

Stress on Blood Vessels: Extra fluid increases the volume of blood passing through your blood vessels, placing extra strain on them. Over time, this leads to high blood pressure, which puts additional strain on your kidneys.

Swelling & Discomfort: With less efficient kidneys in Stage 3, excess fluid can build up, causing swelling in your feet, ankles, or hands. It can leave you feeling bloated and uncomfortable.

Heart Strain: High blood pressure is a major risk factor for heart disease, and your kidneys and heart health are closely linked. So, reducing salt is a win-win!

How Much is Too Much?

The recommended daily salt intake for most adults should be less than 2,300mg of sodium. With Stage 3 kidney disease, your doctor or dietitian might recommend an even lower limit. Don't worry, this doesn't mean your food has to be bland!

Tips To Shake off the Salt Habit

- **Become a Label Detective:** Processed foods and restaurant meals are huge sources of hidden salt. Start reading food labels and comparing brands to find lower-sodium choices.

- **Flavor Boosters:** Herbs, spices, garlic, onions, and citrus zest add lots of flavor without the need for any salt.

- **Cook at Home:** When you prepare your own meals, you have full control over the salt shaker.

- **Rethink Seasoning Blends:** Many packaged spice mixes contain salt. Opt for salt-free versions or make your own!

- **Gradually Reduce It:** If cutting back drastically seems overwhelming, start small. Even slight reductions make a difference over time, and your taste buds will adjust.

Swap This for That: Examples

- Choose low-sodium soups instead of canned ones, or even better, prepare a tasty homemade soup.
- Try freshly roasted chicken, turkey, or fish instead of deli meats and hotdogs.
- Opt for unsalted nuts and seeds, air-popped popcorn, or fresh fruits and vegetables in place of salty chips and snacks.
- Try making your favorite restaurant dishes at home using less salt instead of dining out.

What to Know About Potassium

Potassium is an important mineral with many beneficial roles for the body. It helps to sustain a regular heartbeat and aids the healthy function of your nerves and muscles. However, when an individual has stage 3 kidney disease, potassium can be a problem when it becomes too low or too high in the blood. Therefore, it becomes very critical to manage the potassium level in your blood for your overall health.

Why Potassium Matters in Stage 3 CKD

- **Heart Health:** Potassium helps regulate your heartbeat. Having levels too high (hyperkalemia) or too low (hypokalemia) can lead to irregular heartbeats and chest palpitations and increase the risk of serious heart complications.

- **Muscle Function:** Too high or too low potassium levels can disrupt muscle function, causing weakness, cramps, or even temporary paralysis in severe cases.

- **Nerve Health:** Potassium plays a role in nerve signaling. Changes in levels can lead to tingling, numbness, or changes in sensation.

- **Overall Well-being:** Potassium balance is connected to energy levels, digestion, and how you feel in general.

How Much is Recommended?

The recommended daily intake level for potassium among seniors is between 2000 and 4000mg.

Potassium-Smart Food Choices

The key is to choose a variety of foods with a moderate amount of potassium. Here's a general idea:

- **Lower-Potassium Fruits & Veggies:** Choices like berries, apples, carrots, cucumbers, and cauliflower are kidney-friendly.

- **Leaching:** This method cooks vegetables in water, draining some of the potassium away. It's helpful for higher-potassium options like potatoes.

- **Portion Control:** Even lower-potassium foods should be eaten in moderation. Enjoy a variety with smaller portions of the higher-potassium options.

Phosphorus Management

Phosphorus is a mineral found in many foods. The body needs phosphorus for healthy bones and teeth, cell function, and many other essential processes. However, when you have Stage 3 kidney disease, having too much phosphorus in your blood can create problems.

Why Phosphorus Matters

- **Strong Bones & Teeth:** Most of the phosphorus in the body is found in the skeleton. It's essential for bone health, but in Stage 3 CKD, the balance gets tricky.

- **Hormone Control:** Phosphorus plays a role in regulating specific hormones, including one that helps manage calcium levels in your blood.

- **Itchy Skin:** A buildup of phosphorus can cause itchy, uncomfortable skin.

- **Overall Health:** If phosphorus levels are persistently high, it can even have broader effects on your health, like muscle weakness and joint problems.

The Challenge with Stage 3 Kidney Disease

When the kidneys are healthy, they filter extra phosphorus out of your blood. In Stage 3, they're not as efficient at this task. High phosphorus can have two major consequences:

1. **Calcium Complications:** High phosphorus can cause the body to pull calcium out of the bones, weakening them over time.

2. **Blood Vessel Issues:** Excess phosphorus can form deposits in the blood vessels, leading to stiffness and increasing the risk of heart disease.

How to Manage Phosphorus

The key is to find the right balance of phosphorus in your diet – not too little and not too much! The recommended daily intake for seniors is 800 to 1000mg.

Here are the basics:

- **Food Choices Matter:** Many foods naturally high in protein (meat, poultry, fish, dairy, nuts) are also significant sources of phosphorus.

- **Phosphorus Additives:** Processed foods often contain phosphorus additives to enhance flavor and texture. Watch those labels closely!

- **Medications Help:** Sometimes, medications called phosphate binders are needed to lower phosphorus levels, taken with meals.

Protein Management for Balance

Protein is a building block of the body, essential for repairing tissues, building muscle, and maintaining a healthy immune system. However, when you have Stage 3 kidney disease, figuring out the right amount of protein can be tricky. Here's why it matters and how to strike the right balance.

Why Protein is Important (Even with Kidney Disease)

- **Strength & Function:** Protein helps your body repair and maintain muscle tissue, which is especially important as we age.

- **Immune Health:** Protein plays a role in keeping your immune system strong, helping you fight off infections.

- **Wound Healing:** If you have any wounds or sores, adequate protein aids in the healing process.

The Kidney Connection

When your kidneys are healthy, they filter waste products created when your body breaks down the protein you eat. In Stage 3, this process isn't as efficient, and too much protein can stress your kidneys further. However, too little protein can lead to:

- Muscle loss and weakness

- Increased risk of infections

- Challenges with wound healing

The Right Balance

The ideal amount of protein for you in Stage 3 CKD is individualized. Your doctor and renal dietitian will consider your body size, activity level, and specific kidney function to create a personalized plan. However, as a general guideline, most adults with Stage 3 CKD aim for 0.6 to 0.8 grams of protein per kilogram (kg) of body weight per day.

For example, if you weigh 150 lbs (68 kg), this translates to roughly 41 to 54 grams of protein per day. Remember, this is a starting point and will be adjusted based on your specific needs.

Focus on Quality Protein Sources

With Stage 3 CKD, the type of protein you choose matters. Here's the scoop:

- **Aim for Plant-Based Often:** Beans, lentils, tofu, and nuts are good protein sources, generally easier on your kidneys.

- **Lean Animal Proteins:** Choose poultry, fish, or eggs more often than red meat.

- **Portion Control:** Moderate your portion sizes, even for kidney-friendly protein sources.

Fluid Balance

Staying hydrated is essential for everyone, but if you have Stage 3 kidney disease, how much fluid you should drink becomes more complex. It's not a one-size-fits-all answer, and finding the right balance is vital for your health and well-being.

Why Fluid Balance Matters in Stage 3 CKD

- **Your Kidneys' Role:** When kidneys are healthy, they fine-tune fluid levels based on your needs. In Stage 3, they might not be able to do this as efficiently.

- **Too Much Fluid:** If your kidneys can't filter out excess fluid, it can build up in your body. This can lead to swelling, put a strain on your heart, and make it harder to breathe.

- **Too Little Fluid:** Dehydration is also a concern. It can worsen kidney function, cause constipation, and make you feel tired or dizzy.

The Personalized Approach

The right amount of fluid for you in Stage 3 CKD depends on several factors, including:

- **Urine Output:** If you're still producing a decent amount of urine, your fluid needs may be closer to normal. However, if urine output decreases, your doctor may recommend limiting fluids.

- **Swelling:** If you experience swelling, especially in your legs, ankles, or feet, restricting fluids might be necessary.

- **Overall Health:** Other conditions, like heart failure, can further influence how much fluid is right for you.

How to Track Your Fluid Intake

Your doctor and dietitian will help you determine your fluid goals and how to monitor them. Here are some tips:

- **Measure It:** Use a measuring cup to track how much liquid you drink throughout the day.

- **What Counts**: Remember that fluids aren't just water. Beverages, soups, ice cream, and even foods like watermelon count towards your fluid intake.

- **Thirst Isn't Always Reliable:** With kidney disease, thirst signals might not be accurate. Stick to your recommended amounts, even if you don't feel thirsty.

Tips for Managing Fluid Intake

If you need to limit fluids, here are some strategies:

- **Small Sips:** Take smaller, more frequent sips instead of large gulps at once.

- **Manage Thirst:** Try sucking on ice chips, frozen grapes, or hard candy.

- **Choose Wisely:** Opt for fluids that count toward your allowance but also quench thirst well, like broths or naturally flavored waters.

Why Dietary Adjustments Are Important

Adhering to these dietary recommendations may seem like a significant change, but always keep in mind that the decisions you make directly affect your health and well-being. Here's why it's worthwhile to do these changes:

- **Preserving Your Kidneys**: By reducing the rate at which kidney disease advances, these dietary changes safeguard and nourish your kidneys.

- **Heart Health Boost:** Eating well for kidney health frequently has positive effects on the heart as well. Greater vitality and a longer, healthier life are associated with a lower risk of heart disease.

- **Managing Other ailments:** Diabetes and high blood pressure are two diseases that many seniors deal with on a daily basis. Diets good for the kidneys frequently aid in the co-management of both diseases.

- **Feeling Your Best:** Less waste products building up, fewer medications, and better fluid balance can significantly improve your day-to-day well-being. You may have less discomfort and greater vitality.

- **Empowerment:** While kidney disease brings challenges, actively participating in your health management through diet gives you the capacity to take charge and thrive.

CHAPTER 3

DESIGNING YOUR KIDNEY-FRIENDLY MEAL PLAN

After exploring the key dietary guidelines for managing Stage 3 kidney disease, you might be wondering how to apply these ideas to your everyday routine. It's one thing to understand what to eat and what to avoid; it's another to put that knowledge into practice every day.

This chapter is all about making it easy and practical. We'll cover meal planning strategies, smart shopping tips, and how to read food labels like a pro. Whether you're preparing a meal for one or for a family, you'll find tools here to create a kidney-friendly plan that fits your lifestyle and satisfies your taste buds.

Meal Planning Made Easy for Seniors

Getting Organized

Start by mapping out your meals for the week. A well-planned menu helps you manage your kidney health proactively, ensuring a balanced intake of important nutrients. Well, let's get started:

- **Small Steps, Big Impact:** Planning even a few meals a week is a great start. Don't feel pressured to overhaul everything at once.

- **Flexibility is Key:** Make use of templates that allow you to swap items based on how you feel, what's fresh, or what you have on hand. For greater flexibility, consider thinking in terms of categories (e.g.; protein + vegetable + starch). For example, a more adaptable alternative might be "Monday: Protein + Veggie Stir-fry + Grain" rather than a template specifying "Monday: Chicken Stir-fry with Rice". This leaves room to swap the type of protein, vegetables, and grain depending on what you have on hand.

- **Favorites with a Twist:** Think about how to adjust your favorite meals to be kidney-friendly. Simple substitutions can make a big difference! For example, try using zucchini noodles as an alternative to traditional pasta in your favorite spaghetti and meatball recipe. Likewise, try making scrambled eggs using low-potassium veggies like onions and peppers instead of a bowl of high-potassium cereal.

- **The Power of Leftovers:** Deliberately cook a little extra for easy, nourishing lunches or dinners throughout the week.

The Balanced Plate Model

To ensure each meal supports your kidney health, try this simple visual:

- **Veggies & Fruits Galore:** Fill half your plate with low-potassium vegetables and fruits like cauliflower, cabbage, apples, and berries. Make a list of the ones you really like and stick to it.

- **Quality Protein:** Protein should make up 25% of your dish. Lean options such as fish, poultry, beans, or tofu are recommended. Be mindful of portion sizes to manage your protein intake.

- **Smart Starches:** Grains or starches with less phosphorus, such as bulgur, rice, or bread prepared with refined flour, can be used to fill the remaining quarter.

Batch Cooking

Prepare meals ahead of time to save time and energy throughout the week. Batch cooking is especially helpful for these kidney-friendly staples:

- **Roasted Veggies:** Roast a big tray for quick additions to meals all week.

- **Soups & Stews:** These freeze well and are perfect for lunch or a light dinner.

- **Cooked Protein:** Grill chicken, bake fish, or simmer a pot of beans to use in salads, sandwiches, or stir-fries.

- **Prepped Snacks:** Individually portioned, washed, and cut-up fruits and vegetables are more likely to get eaten!

If you're batch cooking, clearly label and date all meals before freezing. This helps you track freshness and use older items first. Use freezer-safe containers or bags to preserve quality.

Kidney-Conscious Smart Shopping Tips

Navigating the grocery store with kidney health in mind can feel overwhelming. But you can change the way you shop and become more confident in your ability to make the right decisions with a few easy tips.

Make a List & Stick to It: Before you head to the grocery store, make a list based on your meal plan for the week. This keeps you focused and helps you avoid impulsive purchases that might not be kidney-friendly. Ensure you don't feel pressured by grocery flyers or in-store promotions. Your kidney health is the priority.

Fresh First: Focus on fresh foods whenever possible, as processed foods often contain high levels of sodium, phosphorus, and other additives. When fresh isn't available, look for frozen vegetables and fruits with no added salts or sugars.

Label Literacy: Spend some time learning how to read food labels. Look for items low in sodium and without phosphate additives. This skill is crucial in choosing products that support your kidney health.

Smart Swaps & Strategies

- **Protein Power:** Instead of red meat, try poultry, fish, beans, or lentils more often.

- **Canned Goods Comparison:** If using canned beans or vegetables, rinse them well to lower the sodium content. Look for low-sodium varieties.

- **Dairy Delights:** Unsweetened almond or cashew milk can be an alternative to regular milk.

- **Beyond the Veggie Aisle:** Look for kidney-friendly options like unsalted nuts, whole-grain crackers, and air-popped popcorn.

- **When You're Feeling Overwhelmed:** Ask the grocery store staff for help! They might know which products are lower in sodium or point you to suitable options.

Remember: It takes time to adopt new shopping habits. Start small, celebrate your successes, and don't be afraid to seek assistance from your dietitian or support network.

Label Reading 101

While food labels include vital information, they can be difficult to understand at times. Understanding a few essential aspects helps you to make the best decisions for managing your Stage 3 kidney disease.

Sodium:

If you're trying to cut back on sodium, search for labels that say "no salt added" or "low sodium" (140 mg/serving or fewer). Watch out for hidden sodium sources like baking soda or monosodium glutamate (MSG). If two similar products are both "low sodium", select the one with the lowest percentage of the Daily Value (DV). Remember, less than 5% Daily Value (DV) is considered low.

Potassium

Potassium content is usually not captured on food labels, but if listed, compare products and choose those with lower percentages of DV. Be aware of high-potassium foods and learn to recognize alternatives. When in doubt, go more frequently for lower-potassium fruits (such as grapes, berries, apples) and veggies (such as onions, cauliflower, peppers) more often.

Phosphorus

The key to managing your phosphorus is to steer clear of processed foods and those with phosphate additives. Ingredients with "phos" in the name (like sodium phosphate) are red flags. Focus on fresh as whole, unprocessed foods are naturally lower in phosphorus, making them a safer bet.

Example: Soup Showdown

Consider a comparison between two cans of chicken noodle soup. This is what you should do:

1. **Sodium:** If Soup A contains 500mg sodium per serving and 300mg for soup B, then it's best to choose Soup B.

2. **Potassium:** Not specified, but consider the ingredients. If Soup A uses potatoes (higher in potassium), Soup B should be your go-to choice.

3. **Phosphorus:** Avoid Soup A if it contains "sodium phosphate". Soup B features natural ingredients, making it the kidney-friendly winner.

Example: Breakfast Cereal Check

Many breakfast cereals include significant levels of salt and phosphorus. Let's do a comparison:

- **Cereal A:** contains 200mg of sodium for each serving, and includes an ingredient listing of "disodium phosphate".

- **Cereal B:** contains 50mg sodium for each serving, and made with whole grains and has no added phosphorus.

Although potassium might not be listed, Cereal B wins it for kidney health owing to its lower sodium and absence of phosphate additives.

Beyond the Big Three

While sodium, potassium, and phosphorus are crucial to monitor, don't forget about these other important factors when reading labels:

- **Sugar:** Too much added sugar isn't good for anyone and can especially worsen health issues common with CKD, like diabetes. Look for options with "no added sugars."

- **Protein:** Those with CKD need to find the right protein balance. The label tells you how much protein a serving contains, helping you make choices aligned with your dietitian's recommendations.

- **Fiber:** Fiber is your friend! It promotes gut health and helps manage blood sugar. Opt for high-fibre varieties of cereals, bread, and other grain-based foods when possible.

- **Ingredients Matter:** Shorter ingredient lists with recognizable, whole foods are generally a better bet for your kidneys and overall health.

Remember: Don't get overwhelmed! Choose a few things to focus on at first. As you get more comfortable with label reading, you can start paying attention to these additional details.

CHAPTER 4

FOODS TO ENJOY AND AVOID FOR KIDNEY HEALTH

Foods to Enjoy for Kidney Health

Now that you've learned about the main nutrients to consider while dealing with Stage 3 renal disease, it's time to put that information into action by creating tasty and gratifying meals! This section will walk you through the large range of kidney-friendly meals available. We'll look at the best options in each food group, highlighting flavor and variety. Get ready to discover new favorites and dispel the myth that a kidney-friendly diet is restrictive.

Veggie Vitality: Low-Potassium, Nutrient-Rich Options

Vegetables are an essential component of a healthy diet, particularly for kidney function. Concentrate on kinds that are low in potassium yet great in flavor and nutritional value.

- Leafy greens include spinach, kale, and lettuce.
- Cruciferous Crew: Cabbage, cauliflower, and broccoli (in moderation).
- Root vegetable delights include carrots, onions, and radishes.
- Other star vegetables are bell peppers, cucumbers, zucchini, and green beans.

- Garlic and onions offer flavor without adding sodium or potassium.

How to Use

- Cauliflower is adaptable and may be steamed, mashed, or made into rice as a side dish.
- Use Bell Pepper Power to add crunch and color to salads and stir-fries.
- Cabbage Creations: Add to slaws or sauté with garlic for a delicious side dish.
- Add diversity to your cooking by roasting, stir-frying, grilling, or pureeing soups.
- Add finely chopped vegetables to sauces, casseroles, or smoothies for added nutrients.

Flavorful Fruits: Focusing on Lower Potassium Options

Fruits provide a boost of sweetness, critical nutrients, and natural energy to your diet. While certain fruits contain more potassium, there is still a tasty selection to enjoy with Stage 3 renal disease!

Focus on These Favorites:

- **Apples and pears:** Ideal for snacking or baked into desserts.
- **Berries:** Strawberries, raspberries, and blueberries are low in potassium and high in antioxidants. They are Ideal for breakfast or as a dessert topping!

- **Pineapple:** has a tropical taste and is lower in potassium than many other fruits. Ideal for fruit salads or as a or as a zesty ingredient in meals.

- **Citrus:** oranges, limes, and lemons (moderate consumption).

Protein Options: Lean Meats, Fish, and Plant-Based Sources

Protein is necessary for tissue growth and repair, but with Stage 3 renal disease, it is critical to pick judiciously. The good news is that there are many tasty and kidney-friendly protein choices available!

Focus on Lean & Low Potassium

- **Poultry:** Skinless chicken and turkey breast are great options. Try them grilled, baked, or in stir-fried.

- **Fish:** Choose fatty fish like tuna, salmon, and mackerel, which are rich in healthy omega-3 fats. Choose low-mercury choices, with baked or grilled methods being kidney-friendly.

- **Eggs:** Consume them in moderation, depending on the recommended amount by your dietitian.

- **Plant Power:** Beans, lentils, chickpeas, and tofu are excellent for salads, soups, or main dishes. They offer protein, fiber, and a lower-potassium alternative to some meats.

Tips for Success

- **Variety is Key:** Don't get stuck on the same proteins. Mixing it up keeps things interesting and provides a broader range of nutrients.

- **Prep Ahead:** Cook a batch of protein to use throughout the week in salads, stir-fries, or sandwiches.

- **Get Creative:** Experiment with different spices, marinades, and cooking methods to add flavor.

Wholesome Grains & Starches: Kidney-Friendly Selections

Grains and starches are staples in many diets; they supply both energy and vital nutrients. However, with Stage 3 CKD, it is quite important to make mindful choices in this.

Understanding Your Options

- **Whole Grains:** Brown rice, quinoa, whole-wheat bread, and oats offer fiber and nutrients but may need to be enjoyed in moderation. Talk to your dietitian about what's right for you.

- **Less Refined Alternatives:** White rice, white pasta, breads and rolls made from refined white flour are often lower in phosphorus and potassium, making them viable choices. Always check labels for additives.

- **Beyond the Ordinary:** Experiment with Bulgur, couscous, and polenta to add delicious variety and broaden your nutritional intake.

Tips for Success

- **Read Labels:** Look for "whole grain" as the first ingredient if choosing those, and compare sodium and phosphorus content between products, if listed.

- **Portion Control:** Even with healthier choices, it's important to stick to recommended serving sizes.

Experiment: Explore different ways to prepare grains to keep things interesting. Try a new recipe with quinoa or a simple white rice pilaf with herbs.

Dairy Alternatives: Managing Phosphorus Intake

Dairy products provide calcium, but they can also include phosphorus. Finding tasty and kidney-friendly alternatives can be quite beneficial in Stage 3 CKD.

Explore These Options

- **Non-Dairy Milk:** Rice milk, almond milk, soy milk, and other plant-based options are commonly available. Choose unsweetened varieties and look for those fortified with calcium and vitamin D.

- **Plant-Based Yogurt & Cheeses:** These alternatives offer versatility in your cooking and snacking. Experiment with different brands and flavors to find the ones you like.

- **Creamy Substitutions:** Cashew cream or blended silken tofu can be used in recipes as a replacement for heavy cream or sour cream.

- **Non-dairy creamers:** Can add richness and flavor to your coffee or tea.

<u>Tips for Making the Switch</u>

- **Start Slowly:** Try replacing one dairy product at a time to adjust your taste buds gradually.

- **Read Labels:** Look for "unsweetened" options, and check for added phosphorus as some brands contain it.

- **Flavor Boosters:** Herbs, spices, and a touch of lemon can brighten up plant-based alternatives.

- **Don't Be Afraid to Experiment:** There's a whole world of dairy-free recipes out there! Discover new favorites.

Foods to Limit or Avoid

As important as knowing which foods to eat while managing Stage 3 kidney disease is knowing what to limit or avoid when it comes to safeguarding your kidneys and general health. This section will walk you through the many kinds of foods that might cause problems and provide helpful advice on how to steer clear of typical errors and choose healthier foods.

Steering Clear of Sodium Sources

Because high sodium consumption can raise blood pressure and cause fluid retention, it is often concerning for kidney health. Here's how to spot things to stay away from:

- **Processed and pre-packaged foods:** for flavor and preservation, these foods are frequently highly salted. Therefore, cut back on the number of canned soups, freezer meals, and snacks. Instead, go for whole grains, lean meats, and fresh or frozen vegetables.

- **Restaurants Meals:** Eating out might be difficult because a lot of restaurant food contains high amounts of salt. When dining out, request that your food be prepared with less salt; instead, choose simpler alternatives like grilled or steamed foods, where you may customize the sauces and seasoning.

- **Sneaky Sources:** Salad dressings, barbecue sauce, and soy sauce are examples of condiments that are rich in salt. Choose low-sodium or homemade varieties to help manage your consumption. Herbs, spices, and lemon juice are other options for flavoring food without adding too much salt.

Potassium in Moderation

Even though potassium is a necessary mineral, people with Stage 3 kidney disease should be very mindful of how much they consume. An excessive amount of potassium can accumulate in the blood and cause hyperkalemia, a condition that can interfere with heart rhythm. But finding the ideal mix is crucial—you don't want to totally cut off potassium!

These foods are still nutritious but should be enjoyed in smaller portions or less frequently:

- **High-Potassium Fruits and Vegetables:** Consume less of these; oranges, potatoes, tomatoes, and bananas. Rather, opt for lower-potassium substitutes such as bell peppers, berries, and apples.

- **Whole Grains:** Some whole grains contain high amount in potassium. So, watch your portion sizes and choose refined grains such as white bread and white rice where suitable, particularly if your dietitian endorses it.

- **Other Sources:** Lentils, chocolate, beans, nuts, and milk are additional sources of potassium.

Phosphorus Control: Smart Choices with Dairy & Protein Sources

Overdosing on phosphorus can eventually weaken bones and destroy blood vessels over time. Although phosphorus is present in a wide variety of meals, selecting dairy and protein wisely can have a significant impact.

Focus on These Areas

- **Dairy Products:** Phosphorus is found in cheese, yogurt, and milk. Select fewer, smaller servings more often, or look at lower-phosphorus dairy substitutes like rice or almond milk.

- **Proteins and Meats:** Protein-rich foods including meat, chicken, fish, beans, and lentils are also good sources of phosphorus. When it comes to meats, opt for lean cuts wherever feasible and avoid organ meats in particular because they are particularly high in phosphorus. Cooking your meat by boiling or grilling will help to reduce some phosphorus content. As always, adhere to the recommended serving sizes; as a general guideline, one serving should be around the size of your palm.

- **Seafood**: Due to their high phosphorus content, certain types of seafood should be avoided or consumed in moderation:

  o Shellfish with a higher phosphorus level, such mussels, oysters, and scallops, should be consumed in moderation.

  o Crustaceans like crabs and lobsters should be consumed sparingly as they are also high in phosphorus.

  o Fatty fish, while beneficial for their omega-3 fatty acids, can be high in phosphorus too. Fish like salmon, mackerel, and halibut should be consumed in moderation, particularly if you need to keep a careful eye on your phosphorus levels.

Although controlling sodium, potassium, phosphorus, and fluids might seem complicated, being aware of these crucial factors helps you take charge of your diet and your health. Keep in mind that you don't have to give up tasty and filling meals because of the items you restrict or avoid.

You now have the information necessary to manage your Stage 3 renal disease diet with confidence after reading this chapter. Never forget that your dietitian is your most valuable ally during your trip. Never be afraid to seek advice, ask questions, and collaborate to develop a customized strategy that promotes both your love of eating and your health

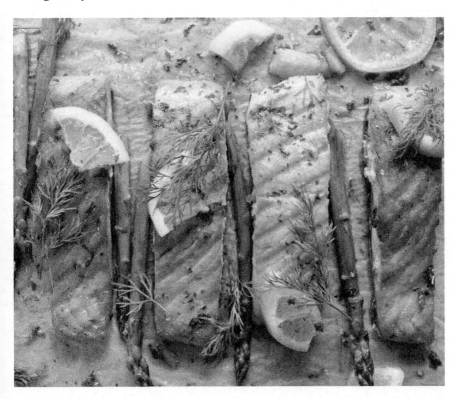

CHAPTER 5

BREAKFAST RECIPES

Apple Cinnamon Oatmeal

Prep Time: 5 mins | Cook Time: 10 mins | Servings: 1

Ingredients:

- 1/2 cup rolled oats
- 1 medium apple, peeled and chopped
- 1/2 tbsp cinnamon
- 1 tbsp honey
- 1 cup water or low-potassium milk alternative (e.g., rice milk)

Directions:

1. In a small saucepan, bring the water or rice milk to a boil.
2. Toss in the rolled oats and chopped apple; gently give it a quick stir.
3. Turn down the heat and let it simmer for approximately 5-10 minutes or until the oats are soft and fully cooked.
4. Take away from heat and stir in the cinnamon and honey.
5. Let it sit for some minutes to thicken up before serving.

Nutritional Information:

Calories: 215 Protein: 3g Sodium: 10mg Fiber: 4g Potassium: 150mg Phosphorus: 95mg Carbs: 45g

Creamy Rice Pudding

Prep Time: 5 mins | Cook Time: 25 mins | Servings: 1

Ingredients:

- ¼ cup white rice
- 1 cup water
- ½ cup rice milk (or low-potassium alternative)
- ½ tbsp vanilla extract
- 1 tbsp sugar (or substitute)
- Pinch of cinnamon (optional)

Directions:

1. Wash the white rice until the water runs clear.
2. In a small saucepan, combine the rinsed rice and 1 cup of water. Bring to a boil.
3. Turn down the heat, cover, and simmer for about 15 minutes or until the rice is tender.
4. Pour the rice milk and sugar into the cooked rice. Give it a good stir.
5. Increase the heat to medium and cook for an extra 10 minutes, stirring frequently until the mixture thickens to your desired consistency.
6. Take it off the heat and stir in vanilla extract. Sprinkle with a pinch of cinnamon if desired.
7. Serve warm for a comforting breakfast or chill in the refrigerator to enjoy cold.

Nutritional Information:

Calories: 215 Protein: 4g Sodium: 30mg Fiber: 1g Potassium: 85mg

Phosphorus: 69mg Carbs: 47g

Vegetable Omelet

Prep Time: 5 mins | Cook Time: 10 mins | Servings: 1

Ingredients:

- 2 egg whites
- 1/4 cup chopped bell peppers (red or green)

- 1/4 cup diced onions
- 1/4 cup diced mushrooms
- 1 tbsp olive oil
- Salt-free seasoning to taste
- Fresh herbs (such as parsley or chives) for garnish

Directions:

1. Over medium heat, heat the olive oil in a non-stick skillet.
2. Toss in the diced onions and bell peppers to the skillet, sautéing until soft.
3. Add mushrooms and cook for an extra 2-3 minutes until all vegetables are soft and lightly browned.
4. In a bowl, whisk the egg whites with salt-free seasoning.
5. Pour the egg whites over the vegetables in the skillet, tilting the pan to ensure an even spread.
6. Cook for approximately 3-4 minutes or until the edges start to lift from the pan. Fold the omelet in half using a spatula.
7. Transfer to a plate, garnish with fresh herbs, and serve immediately.

Nutritional Information:

Calories: 180 Protein: 8g Sodium: 75mg Fiber: 2g Potassium: 210mg Phosphorus: 110mg Carbs: 8g

Cottage Cheese with Pineapple

Prep Time: 2 mins | Cook Time: 0 mins | Servings: 1

Ingredients:

- ½ cup low-sodium cottage cheese
- ½ cup pineapple chunks (fresh or canned in juice)
- 1 tbsp honey or sprinkle of cinnamon (optional)

Directions:

1. If using canned pineapple, drain the pineapple chunks thoroughly.
2. In a small basin, mix the cottage cheese with the pineapple chunks.
3. Drizzle with honey or sprinkle with cinnamon if needed.
4. Stir gently to mix and serve immediately.

Nutritional Information:

Calories: 145 Protein: 14g Sodium: 125mg Fiber: 1g Potassium: 180mg Phosphorus: 120mg Carbs: 15g

Baked Apple Oatmeal

Prep Time: 10 minutes | Cook Time: 25 minutes | Servings: 1

Ingredients:

- 1/2 cup rolled oats
- 1/2 cup unsweetened almond milk
- 1 small apple, peeled and diced
- 1/4 tbsp ground cinnamon
- 1 tbsp chopped walnuts
- 1 tbsp honey or maple syrup (optional)

Directions:

1. Preheat the oven to 350°F (175°C).
2. In an oven-safe dish, mix the rolled oats, cinnamon, diced apple and almond milk.
3. Bake for 20-25 minutes until the oats are tender and the apple is soft.
4. Take out from the oven and garnish with chopped walnuts and a drizzle of honey or maple syrup.
5. Serve warm and enjoy your cozy baked apple oatmeal!

Nutritional Information (per serving):

Calories: 250 Protein: 6g Carbohydrates: 45g Fiber: 7g Sodium: 50mg Potassium: 300mg Phosphorus: 150mg

Zucchini Bread

Prep Time: 15 minutes Cook Time: 1 hour Servings: 16 slices

Ingredients:

- 3 eggs
- 1½ cups sugar
- 1 cup unsweetened applesauce
- 2 cups unpeeled zucchini, shredded
- 1 tbsp vanilla extract
- 2 cups flour
- ¼ tbsp baking powder
- 1 tbsp baking soda
- 1 tbsp cinnamon
- ½ tbsp ginger
- 1 cup unsalted chopped nuts (optional)

Directions:

1. Preheat the oven to a temperature of 375°F (190°C).
2. Beat the eggs in a big bowl.
3. Mix in the applesauce, vanilla extract, shredded zucchini, and sugar.
4. In another bowl, sift flour, baking powder, baking soda, cinnamon, and ginger.
5. Fold the dry ingredients into the egg mixture just until blended (do not overmix).
6. Pour the batter into a loaf pan.
7. Bake for 1 hour or until a toothpick inserted into the center comes out clean.
8. Let the bread cool, then cut it into 16 slices.

Nutritional Information (per slice):

Calories: 200 Carbohydrates: 33.2g Fiber: 2.6g Protein: 4.4g

Sodium: 100mg Potassium: 128mg Phosphorus: 78mg

Quinoa Breakfast Bowl

Prep Time: 5 minutes Cook Time: 15 minutes Servings: 1

Ingredients:

- ½ cup cooked quinoa
- ¼ cup unsweetened almond milk
- ½ tbsp vanilla extract
- ¼ tbsp ground cinnamon
- 1 small apple, diced
- 1 tbsp chopped walnuts
- 1 tbsp honey/maple syrup (optional)

Directions:

1. Mix the cooked quinoa, almond milk, vanilla extract, and cinnamon in a bowl.
2. Heat the mixture in the microwave or on the stovetop.
3. Garnish with diced apple and walnuts. Drizzle honey or maple syrup if desired.
4. Serve warm and enjoy your nutritious quinoa breakfast bowl!

Nutritional Information (per serving):

Calories: 250 Protein: 6g Carbohydrates: 45g Fiber: 6g Sodium: 50 mg Potassium: 300 mg Phosphorus: 150 mg

Vegetable Frittata

Prep Time: 10 minutes Cook Time: 20 minutes Servings: 1

Ingredients:

- 2 eggs

- 1/4 cup red bell pepper, diced
- 1/4 cup green bell pepper, diced
- 1/4 cup zucchini, chopped
- 1/4 cup carrot, chopped
- 1/4 tbsp ground cumin
- A pinch of Salt(if required)/ salt-free spice
- Pepper to taste
- 1 teaspoon olive oil

Directions:

1. Over medium-high heat, heat the olive oil in a sauté pan.
2. Pour in the diced red and green bell peppers, carrot and zucchini. Sauté for about until softened.
3. In a bowl, whisk the eggs with ground cumin, salt(optional), and pepper.
4. Pour the egg mixture over the sautéed vegetables in the pan.
5. Cook for approximately 15 minutes on low to medium heat until the eggs are set and the frittata is a bit golden.
6. Serve warm.

Nutritional Information (per serving):

Calories: 180 Protein: 12g Carbohydrates: 10g Fiber: 2g Sodium: 150 mg Potassium: 200 mg Phosphorus: 120 mg

Peach Compote Toast

Prep Time: 5 mins | Cook Time: 10 mins | Servings: 1

Ingredients:

- 1 slice low-sodium white bread
- ½ cup fresh/frozen peach slices
- 1 tbsp sugar (or substitute)
- ¼ tbsp cinnamon

Directions:

1. Toast the bread slice to your liking.
2. In a small saucepan, combine peach slices, cinnamon, and sugar.
3. Cook for about 10 minutes over medium heat until the peaches are soft and the mixture has thickened into a compote.
4. Spread the warm peach compote over the toasted bread and serve immediately.

Nutritional Information:

Calories: 135 Protein: 2g Sodium: 120mg Fiber: 2g Potassium: 190mg Phosphorus: 40mg Carbs: 28g

Easy Chia Seed Pudding

Prep Time: 5 minutes Time: 4 hours (+chilling time) Servings: 4

Ingredients:

- ½ cup chia seeds
- 1 tbsp vanilla extract
- ¼ cup maple syrup
- ¼ tbsp ground cinnamon
- 1 ½ cups rice milk (low potassium & phosphorus)

Directions:

1. In a bowl or mason jar, combine the chia seeds, vanilla extract, maple syrup, cinnamon, and rice milk.
2. Stir the chia seed blend until well mixed, ensuring the chia seeds don't stick on the sides of the container.
3. Cover the bowl or jar and refrigerate for at least 4 hours or overnight.
4. Add your favorite fresh fruit before serving, if you so desire.

Nutritional Information (per serving):

Calories: 206 Carbohydrates: 32g Protein: 4g Fat: 7g Sodium: 40mg Potassium: 134mg Phosphorus: 78mg Fiber: 7g

Bulgur Wheat Porridge

Prep Time: 5 mins | Cook Time: 15 mins | Servings: 1

Ingredients:

- ¼ cup bulgur wheat
- 1 cup water
- 1 tbsp honey/maple syrup
- Pinch of cinnamon
- ¼ cup chopped apples (optional)

Directions:

1. Add some water in a small saucepan and bring to a boil.
2. Add the bulgur wheat and reduce the heat to a simmer.
3. Cook for approximately 12-15 minutes until the bulgur is soft and the water is absorbed.
4. Stir in honey or maple syrup and a bit of cinnamon for flavor.
5. Mix in chopped apples if desired, and serve warm.

Nutritional Information:

Calories: 190 Protein: 4g Sodium: 10mg Fiber: 4g Potassium: 125mg Phosphorus: 80mg Carbs: 41g

Spicy Tofu Scrambler

Prep Time: 5 minutes Cook Time: 20 minutes Servings: 1

Ingredients:

- 1 clove garlic, minced
- 1/4 cup red bell pepper, diced

- 1/4 cup green bell pepper, diced
- 1/2 cup crumbled tofu
- 1/4 tbsp ground cumin
- A pinch of turmeric (for color)
- A pinch of Salt (if required)/ salt-free spice
- Pepper to taste
- 1 tbsp olive oil

Directions:

1. In a medium-sized, nonstick skillet, sauté the minced garlic and both bell peppers in olive oil.
2. Rinse and drain the tofu, then smash it into the skillet.
3. Add the ground cumin, a pinch of turmeric, salt(optional), and pepper. Stir well.
4. Cook for about 20 minutes on low to medium heat until the tofu turns a slight golden brown.
5. Serve your flavorful tofu scrambler warm.

Nutritional Information (per serving):

Calories: 150 Protein: 12g Carbohydrates: 6g Fiber: 2g Sodium: 100mg Potassium: 180mg Phosphorus: 120mg

Cherry Almond Chia Pudding

Prep Time: 5 minutes Total Time: 4 hours (+ chilling time) Servings: 4

Ingredients:

- ½ cup chia seeds
- 1 ½ cups unsweetened vanilla almond & coconut milk (check for phosphorus additives)
- 1 tbsp vanilla extract
- 2 tbsp maple syrup
- ¼ tbsp cinnamon (optional)

- 2 cups cherries (defrosted if frozen)
- Sliced almonds

Directions:

1. In a mason jar, mix the chia seeds, vanilla extract, almond-coconut milk, maple syrup, and optional cinnamon. Stir well.
2. Cover and refrigerate for not less than 4 hours or overnight.
3. Blend 2 cups of cherries with a little coconut milk until smooth.
4. Layer the chia pudding with the cherry mixture in serving glasses.
5. Top with sliced almonds.

Nutritional Information (per serving):

Calories: 168   Carbohydrates: 14g   Protein: 7g   Sodium: 45mg

Potassium: 271mg Phosphorus: 197mg

Avocado Toast

Prep Time: 5 minutes Servings: 1

Ingredients:

- 1 slice whole-grain bread
- 1/4 ripe avocado
- A pinch of Salt(if required)/ salt-free spice
- Black pepper
- 1 egg (scrambled or poached)
- 1/4 cup halved grape tomatoes
- 1/4 cup arugula
- 1 tbsp balsamic drizzle (voluntary)

Directions:

1. Toast the bread until golden and crispy.
2. Mash the avocado over the toast and sprinkle with salt(optional) and pepper.

3. Top with the cooked egg, halved grape tomatoes, and arugula.
4. Drizzle with balsamic if desired.

Nutritional Information (per serving):

Calories: 249 kcal Carbohydrates: 14g Fiber: 5g Protein: 12g
Sodium: 313mg Potassium: 470mg Phosphorus: 197mg

Low-Sodium Pancakes

Prep Time: 10 minutes Cook Time: 10 minutes Servings: 4 (adjust as needed)

Ingredients:

- 1 cup all-purpose flour
- 1tbsp low-sodium baking powder
- 1 tbsp sugar
- 1 egg
- 1 cup unsweetened almond milk
- 1 tbsp vanilla extract
- Cooking spray

Directions:

1. In a mixing bowl, whisk together the flour, baking powder, and sugar.
2. Add the egg, almond milk, and vanilla extract. Mix until well combined.
3. Heat a non-stick skillet or griddle over medium heat and lightly grease with cooking spray or oil.
4. Pour about 1/4 cup of batter onto the skillet for each pancake.
5. Cook until bubbles form on the surface, then flip and cook the other side until golden brown.

6. Serve with your favorite low-sodium toppings like fresh fruit or a drizzle of pure maple syrup.

Nutritional Information (per serving):

Calories: 168 Carbohydrates: 33 g Protein: 5g Fiber: 1g Sodium: 45 mg Potassium: 50 mg Phosphorus: 80 mg

CHAPTER 6

LUNCH RECIPES

Turkey and Cheese Wrap

Prep Time: 10 mins | Cook Time: 0 mins | Servings: 1

Ingredients:

- 1 low-sodium whole wheat wrap
- 2 slices low-sodium turkey breast
- 1 slice low-phosphorus cheese
- ¼ cup shredded lettuce
- 1 tomato slices
- 1 tbsp low-fat mayo/yogurt spread

Directions:

1. Lay your whole wheat wrap down flat on a clean surface.
2. Take your low-fat mayo or yogurt spread and give it a good, even layer all over the wrap.
3. Pile on the turkey slices. Layer them nicely over the spread.
4. Place the cheese slice right on top of the turkey.
5. For some crunch and freshness - add your shredded lettuce and tomato slices on top of the cheese.
6. Carefully roll the wrap tightly, starting from the edge closest to you. Make sure all that yummy filling stays inside.
7. Cut the wrap in half diagonally and enjoy it right away, or if you're packing it for later, wrap it in foil to keep it fresh.

Nutritional Information:

Calories: 280 Protein: 24g Sodium: 320mg Fiber: 3g Potassium: 195mg Phosphorus: 220mg Carbs: 26g

Balsamic Marinated Mushrooms

Prep Time: 15 minutes Cook Time: 2 hours Servings: 3 mushrooms

Ingredients:

- 12 button mushrooms, stems removed
- ¼ cup balsamic vinegar
- ¼ cup apple cider vinegar
- 1 tbsp chopped chive (plus extra for garnish)
- Pinch of freshly ground black pepper

Directions:

1. Toss the mushroom in a medium-sized bowl or Tupperware container
2. Pour in the entire ingredients, from balsamic vinegar, chopped chive, apple cider vinegar to the black pepper
3. Thoroughly mix everything using your hands.
4. Cover the bowl or Tupperware and refrigerate the marinating mushrooms for a minimum of 2 hours (up to a maximum of 2 days). Shake the container occasionally to redistribute the vinegar dressing.
5. When ready to serve:
   - Remove the mushrooms from the bowl or Tupperware, separating them from the vinegar.
   - Sprinkle with extra chopped chives.
   - Optionally, drizzle some of the leftover vinegar on top of the mushrooms or reduce the vinegar in a pot over medium heat to create a thicker sauce.

Nutritional Information (per serving):

Calories: 29 Carbohydrates: 4.7 g Dietary Fiber: 0.6 g Protein: 1.8 g

Sodium: 7.1 mg Potassium: 203 mg Phosphorus: 51.1 mg

Apple Cranberry Walnut Salad

Prep Time: 45 minutes Cook Time:1 hour Servings: 6 servings (½ cup per serving)

Ingredients:

- 2 cups red seedless grapes, halved
- 1⅓ cups chopped walnuts
- 1¼ cups pomegranate-infused dried cranberries
- 4 stalks celery, chopped
- 7 medium Gala apples, cored & sliced
- 8 oz Cranberry Balsamic Dressing

Directions:

1. Begin by preparing the grapes. Rinse a cluster of red grapes thoroughly, then carefully separate the individual grapes from the stem. Using a paring knife, slice each grape in half and place them in a large mixing bowl.
2. Add the chopped walnuts and pomegranate-infused dried cranberries to the bowl with the grapes.
3. Toss the chopped celery and apple into the bowl with the other ingredients.
4. Pour the entire bottle of cranberry dressing over the mixture. Give everything a good stir, ensuring the dressing coats all the ingredients evenly.
5. Cover the bowl and let the salad chill in the refrigerator for at least 2 hours, or up to 2 days. This will allow the flavors to meld beautifully.
6. Once chilled, serve your Apple Cranberry Walnut Salad as a refreshing side dish or a light and satisfying lunch option.

Nutritional Information (per serving):

Calories: 94 Carbohydrates: 15.7g Dietary Fiber: 1.8g Protein: 1g

Sodium: 60.7mg Potassium: 102.6mg Phosphorus: 26.2mg

Baked Salmon with Dill

Prep Time: 5 mins | Cook Time: 10-15 mins | Servings: 1 (with potential for leftovers)

Ingredients:

- 1 (2-3 ounce) salmon fillet
- 1/2 tbsp olive oil
- 1 tbsp fresh dill, chopped
- Lemon slices (for garnish)
- Freshly ground black pepper, to taste

Directions:

1. Preheat your oven to a Fahrenheit degree of 375.
2. Thoroughly rinse the salmon in water and then pat dry it with paper towel
3. Lay out a sheet of aluminum foil on a baking tray and gently place your salmon fillet right in the center.
4. Drizzle olive oil over the salmon, then sprinkle chopped dill and black pepper over it.
5. Carefully wrap it up tight in the foil.
6. Bake for about 10-15 minutes in the preheated oven or until the salmon flakes easily with a fork.
7. Serve hot and enjoy with a garnish of lemon slices.

Nutritional Information (for 2-3 oz serving):

Calories: 200 Protein: 16g Sodium: 60mg Fiber: 0g Potassium: 300mg Phosphorus: 180mg Carbs: 0g

Roasted Asparagus and Wild Mushroom Stew

Prep Time: 45 minutes Cook Time: 30 minutes Servings: 6 servings (⅔ cup per serving)

Ingredients:

- 1 lb. fresh asparagus
- 1 oz. dried wild mushroom medley (such as morels or other varieties)
- 1 cup very hot water
- 2 tbsps olive oil
- 2 celery stalks, diced
- 1 carrot stick, diced
- 1 small onion, diced
- 1 fennel (anise) head, diced
- 4 sprigs fresh thyme
- Pinch of cayenne pepper
- Ground black pepper, to taste
- 1 tbsp dried sage
- 1 tbsp fresh chopped parsley
- 1 tbsp + 1 tbsp dry Marsala wine
- 1 bay leaf
- ⅛ tbsp garlic powder
- ⅛ tbsp onion powder
- 2 cups low-sodium vegetable stock
- 2 oz. pine nuts (for garnish)

Directions:

1. Preheat your oven to a Fahrenheit degree of 400° (200°C).
2. Thoroughly wash and trim the asparagus. Then, spread them out in a single layer on a baking sheet.
3. Lightly mist the asparagus with about a teaspoon of olive oil. Roast in the preheated oven for 10 minutes.

4. Remove the asparagus, allow it to cool and then chop it into bits.
5. Put the mushrooms in a bowl and pour in a cup of hot water. Allow it to soak, and then preserve the water for later use.
6. Heat up a teaspoon of olive oil in a non-stick saucepan over medium-high heat. Toss in the diced celery, carrots, onions, and fennel. Sauté until the onions turn translucent.
7. Stir in the fresh thyme, cayenne pepper, dried sage, chopped parsley, Marsala wine, a bay leaf, and garlic and onion powder. Let that cook for an extra minute, stirring the whole time.
8. Add the veggie stock, the mushroom water, and the rehydrated mushrooms into the saucepan. Stir and allow it to simmer for 15 minutes to blend the flavors together.
9. Arrange the roasted asparagus pieces in the bottom of a serving dish.
10. Pour the mushroom stew over the asparagus.
11. For a lovely crunch and nutty flavor, sprinkle pine nuts atop it.
12. Serve warm and enjoy the Roasted Asparagus and Wild Mushroom Stew.

Nutritional Information (per serving):

Calories: 103 Carbohydrates: 11.7g Dietary Fiber: 3.9g Protein: 3.4g Sodium: 78.8mg Potassium: 436.8mg Phosphorus: 69.8mg

Vegetable Stir-Fry with Tofu

Prep Time: 10 mins | Cook Time: 10 mins | Servings: 2

Ingredients:

- 1/2 block firm tofu, drained and cubed
- 1 cup bell peppers, mixed colors, sliced
- 1/2 cup carrots, julienned

- 1 cup bok choy, chopped
- 2 tbsps low-sodium soy sauce
- 1 tbsp sesame oil
- 1 clove garlic, minced
- 1 tbsp fresh ginger, grated

Directions:

1. Over medium heat, heat sesame oil in a large skillet.
2. Add garlic and ginger, sautéing briefly until fragrant.
3. Add tofu cubes and bake until it becomes lightly golden on each side.
4. Add the bell peppers, carrots, and bok choy to the pan. Stir-fry for approximately 5-7 minutes or until the vegetables are tender-crisp.
5. Drizzle the stir-fry with low-sodium soy sauce and toss to coat all the ingredients evenly.
6. Serve hot and enjoy.

Nutritional Information:

Calories: 200 Protein: 10g Sodium: 150mg Fiber: 3g Potassium: 300mg Phosphorus: 150mg Carbs: 18g

Pasta Primavera

Prep Time: 10 mins | Cook Time: 20 mins | Servings: 2

Ingredients:

- 2 cups cooked whole wheat spaghetti
- 1 cup broccoli, chopped
- 1/2 cup sliced carrots
- 1/2 cup green peas
- 1/2 bell pepper, sliced
- 2 tbsps olive oil

- 2 cloves garlic, minced
- Salt-free Italian seasoning to taste

Directions:

1. Over medium heat, heat the olive oil in a large skillet.
2. Add garlic and sauté for 1 minute.
3. Add carrots, bell pepper, broccoli and peas. Cook for approximately 7-10 minutes until they are tender.
4. Add the cooked spaghetti to the skillet. Then sprinkle Italian seasoning over it. Toss until well combined.
5. Serve warm and enjoy.

Nutritional Information:

Calories: 320 Protein: 10g Sodium: 70mg Fiber: 8g Potassium: 380mg Phosphorus: 180mg Carbs: 55g

Baked Chicken with Lemon and Herbs

Prep Time: 10 minutes Cook Time: Approximately 1 hour (15 minutes per pound) Servings: 4-6 (3-ounce servings)

Ingredients:

- 1 (4-5 pound) whole chicken, fresh or thawed
- 2 tbsps unsalted butter, softened
- 2 1/2 tbsps chopped fresh herbs (like sage, thyme, etc.)
- 2 cloves garlic, peeled and crushed
- 1 small lemon, thinly sliced
- 1 tbsp olive oil

Directions:

1. Preheat your oven to a Fahrenheit degree of 450 (232°C).
2. Put the whole chicken in a roasting pan.

3. In a small bowl, combine some softened butter with the chopped fresh herbs and crushed garlic. Mix it all together until it's well combined.
4. Gently stuff the chicken's cavity with this herbed butter mixture and a few thinly sliced lemons.
5. Drizzle some olive oil over the chicken's skin and rub it in to enhance crisping during roasting.
6. Cook in the oven for about 15 minutes on each pound, or until the internal temperature of the chicken gets to 165°F (74°C), ensuring the skin is golden brown and crispy.
7. Once the chicken is cooked to perfection, carefully drain those buttery juices from the roasting pan and drizzle over the chicken for extra flavor. Garnish with the lemon slices.
8. Allow the chicken to cool for approximately 20 minutes before carving to let the juices redistribute throughout the meat for optimal flavor and moisture.

Nutritional Information (per serving):

Calories: 251 Protein: 19g Sodium: 77mg Dietary Fiber: 0g

Potassium: 222mg Phosphorus: 188mg Carbohydrates: 0g

Baked Turkey Spring Rolls

Prep Time: 20 minutes Cook Time: 25 minutes Servings: 8 spring rolls

Ingredients:

- 20 oz lean ground turkey breast
- 1 tbsp balsamic vinegar
- 1 tbsp sesame oil
- 2 tbsps minced cilantro
- 2 tbsps vegetable oil
- 2½ cups coleslaw mix (shredded cabbage and carrots)

- 2 tbsps ground black pepper
- 16 frozen spring roll pastry wrappers
- Non-stick cooking spray

Directions:

1. Preheat your oven to a Fahrenheit degree of 400 (200°C).
2. Over medium-high heat in a non-stick skillet, cook the ground turkey, minced garlic, and grated ginger, stirring occasionally, until the turkey is cooked through (about 4-5 minutes). Drain thoroughly.
3. Transfer that cooked turkey blend to a bowl and mix in the balsamic vinegar, sesame oil, and minced cilantro. Stir thoroughly until well combined.
4. Spread one spring roll wrapper on a clean surface. Spoon about 2 tablespoons of the turkey blend diagonally across the center of the wrapper; then top with a small amount of coleslaw mix.
5. Carefully fold in the sides of the wrapper and roll it up tightly, same as a burrito. Repeat with the rest of the wrappers and filling until you've used it all up
6. Line a baking sheet with parchment paper and arrange the rolled spring rolls on it. Light spray the rolls with non-stick cooking spray to help them get crispy.
7. Bake in the preheated oven for approximately 20-25 minutes or until they achieve a golden-brown color and a crispy texture
8. Allow the spring rolls to cool slightly before serving. Enjoy them with your preferred dipping sauce, such as sweet chili sauce or soy sauce

Nutritional Information (per spring roll):

Calories: 90 Protein: 8g Sodium: 120mg Dietary Fiber: 1g

Potassium: 140mg Phosphorus: 60mg Carbohydrates: 10g

Mediterranean Quinoa Salad with Roasted Summer Vegetables

Prep Time: 15 minutes Cook Time: 30 minutes (+roasting time)
Servings: 4 servings

Ingredients:

- ⅓ cup uncooked quinoa, rinsed (or 1 cup cooked quinoa)
- 1 small eggplant, diced
- 1 small zucchini, diced
- 1 small yellow squash (or zucchini), diced
- 3 to 4 tbsps olive oil, divided
- A pinch of Salt (if required)/ salt-free spice
- Freshly ground black pepper
- 1 ½ to 2 tbsps lemon juice, to taste
- 1 clove garlic, minced
- 2 tbsps fresh basil leaves, chopped
- 2 tbsps fresh mint leaves, chopped
- 2 tbsps pine nuts, toasted
- For garnish: crumbled feta (optional)

Instructions:

1. Preheat your oven to a Fahrenheit degree of 425 (220°C) and place racks in the top and lower thirds of the oven.
2. Use parchment paper to line two big baking sheets. Evenly divide the diced yellow squash, zucchini, and eggplant among the sheets. Pour in one tablespoon of olive oil and stir to ensure uniform coating.
3. Line two large, rimmed baking sheets with parchment paper. Spread diced eggplant, zucchini, and yellow squash evenly between the sheets. Drizzle them with a tablespoon of olive oil and give it a good toss to ensure it's all coated.
4. Add salt(optional) and pepper for seasoning. Roast for 20-30 minutes until softened and lightly browned. Set aside to cool.

5. To make the quinoa, put the raw quinoa in a small saucepan and add ⅔ cup of water. Bring to a boil, lower the heat to a simmer, cover, and allow the quinoa to cook for approximately 15 minutes or until it is tender and the water has been completely absorbed. When the quinoa is done, fluff it with a fork.

6. Make the dressing by mixing together olive oil, lemon juice, minced garlic, salt, and pepper in a small bowl.

7. In a large bowl, mix the cooked quinoa, roasted vegetables, and chopped basil and mint. Pour the dressing over everything and gently toss to coat.

8. Garnish with toasted pine nuts and crumbled feta if desired. Serve warm or at room temperature.

Nutritional Information (per serving):

Calories: 250 Protein: 5g Sodium: 120mg Dietary Fiber: 5g Potassium: 250mg Phosphorus: 100mg Carbohydrates: 30g

Mushroom Barley Soup

Prep Time: 15 minutes Cook Time: 40 minutes Servings: 6 servings

Ingredients:

- Extra virgin olive oil
- 1 ½ pounds mixed mushrooms (baby bella & white)
- 1 onion, chopped
- 2-3 cloves garlic, minced
- 2 stalks celery, chopped
- 2 carrots, chopped
- 1 tbsp coriander
- ½ tbsp cumin
- ½ tbsp smoked paprika
- 4 cups vegetable broth

- ½ cup pearl barley
- A pinch of Salt(if required)/ salt-free spice
- Pepper to taste

Instructions:

1. Over medium heat in a large pot, heat the olive oil.
2. Toss in the chopped onions, garlic, celery, and carrots. Cook until soft and fragrant.
3. Add sliced mushrooms and sauté until their moisture is released.
4. Stir in the warm spices (coriander, cumin, and smoked paprika), and vegetable broth. Give everything a good mix.
5. Bring the mixture to a gentle simmer, then add the pearl barley.
6. Cook, covered, until barley is soft, approximately 30 minutes.
7. Season with salt(optional) and pepper.
8. Serve hot.

Nutritional Information (per serving):

Calories: 180 kcal Protein: 6g Sodium: 300mg Dietary Fiber: 6g

Potassium: 200mg Phosphorus: 120mg Carbohydrates: 30g

Chicken Tortilla Casserole

Prep Time: 20 minutes Cook Time: 35 minutes Servings: 8 servings

Ingredients:

- 1/2 medium onion, chopped
- 2 cloves garlic, minced
- 1 tbsp vegetable oil
- 1/2 tbsp dried cumin
- 1/2 tbsp dried oregano
- 1/4 tbsp black pepper

- 1/4 cup low-sodium canned green chiles, diced
- 1 (10.75 oz) can reduced-sodium cream of chicken soup
- 1 (10.75 oz) can reduced-sodium cream of mushroom soup
- 1 cup low-sodium chicken broth
- 6 corn tortillas, cut into quarters
- 1/2 cup shredded low-fat cheese (cheddar or Monterey Jack)
- 2 cups cooked chicken, shredded or diced

Instructions:

1. Sauté onion and garlic in vegetable oil in a large skillet over medium heat until softened.
2. Add cumin, oregano, and black pepper. Cook for another minute, stirring constantly.
3. Stir in green chiles, cream of chicken soup, mushroom soup, and chicken broth. Bring to a simmer.
4. In a 9x13-inch baking dish, layer corn tortillas, chicken, sauce, and cheese.
5. Repeat layers until all ingredients are used, ending with cheese on top.
6. Bake at 375°F (190°C) for 25-30 minutes or until bubbly and golden brown.
7. Let cool slightly before serving.

Nutritional Information (per serving):

Calories: 280 Protein: 15g Sodium: 550mg Dietary Fiber: 3g Potassium: 320mg Phosphorus: 180mg Carbohydrates: 25g

Zucchini Tortilla Bites

Prep Time: 10 minutes Cook Time: 15 minutes Servings: Approx 4 servings (adjust as needed)

Ingredients:

- 2 corn tortillas, cut into triangles

- 2 tbsps vegetable oil
- 1 zucchini, peeled into ribbons/noodles
- 1 cup arugula, rinsed
- Juice and zest of 1 lime
- 2 tbsps fresh cilantro, chopped
- Pinch of red chili pepper flakes (optional)

Directions:

1. Preheat the oven to a Fahrenheit degree of 375 (190°C).
2. Brush the triangles of corn tortillas with vegetable oil.
3. Spread them out on a baking sheet and bake in the oven for approximately 10-12 minutes or until they become crispy.
4. Combine the zucchini ribbons with the zest and juice of the lime in a separate dish.
5. Top the cooked tortilla triangles with arugula and zucchini ribbons.
6. Add some chopped cilantro and a dash of red chili flakes as garnish.
7. Serve warm as a delightful appetizer or snack.

Nutritional Information (per serving):

Calories: 120 kcal Protein: 2g Sodium: 80mg Dietary Fiber: 2g

Potassium: 250mg Phosphorus: 40mg Carbohydrates: 20g

Tropical Chicken Risotto

Prep Time: 45 minutes Cook Time: 45 minutes Servings: Approx 4 servings (adjust as needed)

Ingredients:

- 1 cup cooked basmati rice
- 1 fillet of chicken breast
- 8 tbsps frozen green peas

- ¼ cup chopped red bell pepper
- 3 cloves of chopped garlic
- 4 tbsps chopped onion
- 1 tbsp blanched almonds
- 1 tbsp chopped parsley
- 1 tbsp ground cumin
- 1 tbsp seedless black raisins
- 2 tbsps canola oil
- Juice of ½ lime

Directions:

1. Slice the red bell pepper into thin strips and keep aside.
2. Cook the basmati rice as per package instructions for 1 cup of cooked rice.
3. Boil the green peas in water and drain. Season with lime juice chopped red bell pepper, and 1 clove of chopped garlic.
4. Heat a tablespoon of oil in a pan over medium heat. Sauté a clove of chopped garlic and two tablespoons of chopped onion until fragrant,
5. Add the chicken breast into the pan, as well as the ground cumin and chopped parsley. Cook until the chicken is done.
6. Add the cooked rice to the pan. Sauté it, adding a splash of water if needed to help it warm through
7. Mix the chicken, red bell pepper, and seasoned peas with the cooked rice.
8. Sprinkle blanched almonds and raisins over the risotto.
9. Serve warm and enjoy this tropical-inspired dish!

Nutritional Information (per serving):

Calories: 367 kcal Protein: 19.2g Sodium: 93mg Dietary Fiber: 3.9g

Potassium: 381mg Phosphorus: 186 mg Carbohydrates: 35.7g

Chipotle Shrimp Tacos Recipe

Prep Time: 10 minutes Cook Time: 15 minutes Servings: Approx 4 servings (adjust as needed)

Ingredients:

- 1 lb large shrimp, peeled & deveined
- 2 tbsp Mazola® Corn Oil
- 1 tbsp onion powder
- 1 tbsp garlic powder
- 1 tbsp soy sauce
- 1-2 canned chipotle peppers in adobo sauce
- Corn tortillas
- Cabbage slaw (made with shredded cabbage, lime juice, and cilantro)
- Lime wedges
- Avocado slices (optional)

Directions:

1. Put the peeled shrimp, soy sauce, and onion and garlic powders in a bowl. Toss to coat.
2. Put a skillet over medium heat and heat the Mazola® Corn Oil.
3. Add the marinated shrimp to the skillet. Cook for approximately 2-3 minutes per side or until done.
4. While cooking the shrimp, finely chop up the amount of chipotle peppers you want from the can - based on how spicy you like things.
5. Once the shrimp is done, toss in the chopped chipotle peppers and a spoonful of smoky adobo sauce. Stir to combine everything.
6. Reheat your corn tortillas.

7. Assemble the tacos: Place a few shrimp on each tortilla, top with cabbage slaw, and garnish with lime wedges and avocado slices.
8. Serve right away and savor your tasty tacos with chipotle shrimp.

Nutritional Information (per serving):

Calories: 250 kcal Protein: 20g Sodium: 450mg Dietary Fiber: 3g

Potassium: 350mg Phosphorus: 180mg Carbohydrates: 20g

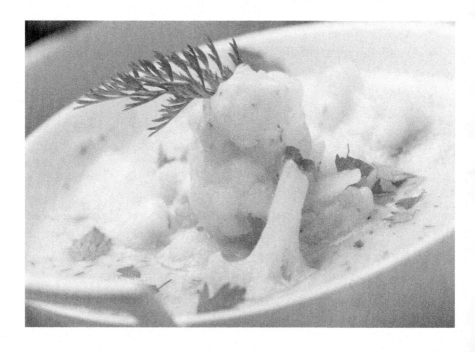

CHAPTER 7

DINNER

Lemon Herb Grilled Salmon

Prep Time: 15 minutes Cook Time: 10 minutes Servings: 4

Ingredients:

- 4 salmon fillets (about 6 oz each)
- 2 tbsps olive oil
- Juice of 1 lemon
- 2 cloves garlic, minced
- 1 tbsp dried thyme
- 1 tbsp dried rosemary
- A pinch of Salt(if required)/ salt-free spice
- Pepper to taste
- Lemon wedges for garnish

Directions:

1. Over a medium-high heat, preheat the grill.
2. Mix the olive oil, lemon juice, minced garlic, dried thyme, dried rosemary, salt(optional), and pepper in a small bowl.
3. Put the salmon pieces in a shallow dish and empty the marinade over them. Allow it to sit for approximately 10 minutes.
4. Take the salmon out of the marinade and throw away the extra liquid.
5. Cook the salmon fillets through and flake readily with a fork after grilling them for around 4–5 minutes on each side.
6. Serve the grilled salmon with lemon wedges on the side.

Nutritional Information (per serving):

Calories: 300 Protein: 34g Sodium: 100mg Fiber: 0g Potassium: 400mg Phosphorus: 400mg Carbohydrates: 1g

Tropical Chicken Risotto:

Prep Time: 20 minutes Cook Time: 55 minutes Servings: 8

Ingredients:

- 13 oz reduced-fat, reduced-sodium cream of chicken soup
- 8 oz plain soy yogurt
- 1 ½ tsp chili powder
- ½ tsp cumin
- 1 large cooked chicken breast, shredded
- 8 small corn tortillas, torn
- ⅓ each: red, yellow, orange bell pepper, chopped
- 3 tbsp fresh cilantro, chopped
- 1 cup sweet yellow corn
- Green chilies
- ½ cup reduced-fat Mexican cheese blend
- ¼ cup unsweetened rice milk

Directions:

1. Preheat the oven to a degree Fahrenheit of 350 (175°C). Drizzle nonstick cooking spray over a 13x9-inch baking dish.
2. Combine together in a large dish the soup, soy yogurt, rice milk, chili powder, cumin, shredded chicken, torn tortillas, bell peppers, and corn.
3. Pour the mixture into the prepared baking dish. Cover it tightly with foil and bake for 40 minutes.
4. Take the casserole out of the oven and remove the foil. Sprinkle ½ cup of reduced-fat cheese over the top.

5. Put it back in the oven, uncovered, for another 5-10 minutes or until the cheese is melted and bubbly.
6. Once done, let the casserole rest for a few minutes. Then, just before serving, sprinkle it with some fresh chopped cilantro for a final touch of flavor and color.

Nutritional Information (per serving):

Calories: 172 Carbohydrates: 4g Protein: 11.1g Fat: 12.4g Sodium: 244.9mg Fiber: 2g Potassium: 284mg Phosphorus: 175.9mg

Cauliflower Rice Stir-Fry

Prep Time: 15 minutes Cook Time: 15 minutes Servings: 4

Ingredients:

- 1 medium head of cauliflower (about 2 lbs)
- 1 tbsp vegetable oil
- 1 medium onion, sliced
- 2 cloves garlic, minced
- 1/2 red bell pepper, sliced
- 1/2 yellow bell pepper, sliced
- 1/2 cup white mushrooms, sliced
- 1 small zucchini, julienned
- 2 tbsps low-sodium soy sauce
- 1 tbsp rice vinegar
- 1 tbsp sesame oil
- 1/2 tbsp ground ginger
- 1/4 tbsp crushed red pepper flakes (adjust to taste)
- 2 green onions, sliced (for garnish)
- Sesame seeds (for garnish)

Directions:

1. Chop the cauliflower into rice-like florets and pulse it in a food processor until they look like little rice grains. Set aside.
2. Heat up some vegetable oil in a large skillet or wok over medium-high heat.
3. Toss in the minced garlic and sliced onion. Sauté until fragrant.
4. Next, add the bell peppers, mushrooms, and zucchini to the pan. Stir-fry everything for about 3-4 minutes, until the veggies are slightly tender.
5. Push the vegetables to one side of the pan and add the cauliflower rice to the other side.
6. In a small bowl, whisk together the soy sauce, rice vinegar, sesame oil, ground ginger, and red pepper flakes. Pour over the cauliflower rice.
7. Stir-fry it all for 3-4 minutes until the cauliflower is cooked through but still somewhat crunchy.
8. Top with sesame seeds and thinly sliced green onions.
9. Serve hot as a main dish or as a side.

Nutritional Information (per serving):

Calories: 115 kcal Protein: 4 g Sodium: 280mg Fiber: 4g Potassium: 320mg Phosphorus: 75mg Carbohydrates: 15g

Quinoa Stuffed Bell Peppers

Prep Time: 20 minutes Cook Time: 30 minutes Servings: 6

Ingredients:

- 3 cups cooked quinoa (rinsed)
- 1 (4-oz) can low-sodium green chiles
- 1 cup corn kernels
- ½ cup low-sodium black beans, rinsed

- ½ cup low-sodium diced tomatoes
- ½ cup low-sodium shredded pepper jack cheese
- ¼ cup crumbled feta cheese
- 3 tbsp chopped cilantro
- 1 tsp each: cumin, garlic powder, onion powder
- ½ tsp chili powder
- A pinch of Salt(if required)/ salt-free spice
- Pepper to taste
- 6 bell peppers, prepared

Directions:

1. Preheat the oven to a degree Fahrenheit of 350 (175°C). Line a 9×13 baking dish with parchment paper.
2. Transfer the cooked quinoa, green chilies, corn, black beans, diced tomatoes, feta and pepper jack cheeses, chopped cilantro, cumin, onion, garlic, and chili powders, as well as salt(optional) and pepper, into a big bowl. Mix well.
3. Spoon the filling into each bell pepper pore.
4. Arrange the filled bell peppers in the baking dish, cavity side up.
5. Bake in the preheated oven for 25-30 minutes or until the peppers are tender and the filling is heated through.
6. Serve immediately.

Nutritional Information (per serving):

Calories: 250 Protein: 10g Sodium: 300mg Fiber: 6g Potassium: 180mg Phosphorus: 150 g Carbohydrates: 35g

Cranberry Pecan Rice Pilaf

Prep Time: 10 minutes Cook Time: 25 minutes Servings: 4

Ingredients:

- 1 cup long-grain white rice
- 2 cups low-sodium vegetable broth
- 1/2 cup dried cranberries
- 1/2 cup chopped pecans
- 1 small onion, finely chopped
- 2 cloves garlic, minced
- 1 tbsp olive oil
- A pinch of Salt(if required)/ salt-free spice
- Pepper to taste
- Fresh parsley for garnish

Directions:

1. Heat the olive oil in a medium saucepan over medium heat. Add the minced garlic and diced onion. Sauté until the onion is translucent.
2. Add the rice to the saucepan and stir to coat it with the flavorful onion and garlic mixture.
3. Add the veggie broth and heat until it boils. Turn the heat down low, cover the saucepan, and let it simmer gently for about 15 minutes.
4. After 15 minutes, stir in the dried cranberries and chopped pecans.
5. Cover the saucepan again and continue simmering for another 10 minutes, or until the rice is tender and all the liquid is absorbed.
6. Season with salt(optional) and pepper to taste.
7. Before serving, fluff the rice with a fork and sprinkle with fresh parsley.

Nutritional Information (per serving):

Calories: 250 Protein: 4g Sodium: 150mg Fiber: 2g Potassium: 120mg Phosphorus: 60mg Carbohydrates: 45g

Chinese-Style Asparagus

Prep Time: 15 minutes Cook Time: 10 minutes Servings: 4

Ingredients:

- 1 bunch fresh asparagus (about 1 lb), trimmed and cut into bite-sized pieces
- 2 cloves garlic, minced
- 1 tbsp low-sodium soy sauce
- 1 tbsp sesame oil
- 1 tbsp vegetable oil
- 1/2 tbsp grated fresh ginger
- Pinch of red pepper flakes (optional)
- Sesame seeds for garnish

Directions:

1. Add water to a pot and bring it to a boil. Toss in the asparagus and let it simmer until slightly tender in about 2 – 3 minutes. Drain and set them aside for a moment.
2. In a skillet over medium heat, preheat the vegetable oil.
3. Toss in the minced garlic and grated ginger. Sauté for 1-2 minutes until fragrant.
4. Pour the blanched asparagus into the skillet.
5. Drizzle with low-sodium soy sauce and sesame oil.
6. Combine all the ingredients to coat the asparagus properly.
7. If desired, sprinkle a pinch of red pepper flakes for a little heat.
8. Stir-fry the asparagus for 3-4 minutes until heated through but still crisp-tender.
9. Transfer the Chinese-style asparagus to a serving dish.
10. Garnish with sesame seeds.

Nutritional Information (per serving):

Calories: 50   Protein: 2g   Sodium: 100mg   Fiber: 2g
Potassium: 150mg Phosphorus: 30mg Carbohydrates: 6g

Broccoli with Garlic and Lemon

Prep Time: 10 minutes Cook Time: 10 minutes Servings: 4

Ingredients:

- 1 lb broccoli florets
- 2 tbsp water
- 4 tsp fresh lemon juice
- 3 tbsp butter
- 2 cloves garlic, minced
- A pinch of Salt(if required)/ salt-free spice
- Pepper to taste

Directions:

1. Add broccoli florets to a large pan and heat it to medium.
2. In a small dish, combine the water and two tablespoons of lemon juice; drizzle the mixture over the broccoli.
3. Cover the skillet and let the broccoli steam until it turns bright green and tender, in about 10 to 15 minutes.
4. Meanwhile, melt butter in a small saucepan over medium-low heat; stir in minced garlic and salt(optional). Reduce heat to low and sauté the garlic until golden brown, about 8 minutes.
5. Once the broccoli is done, drain off any excess liquid and return it to the skillet. Sprinkle the remaining lemon juice over the broccoli and stir in the garlic mixture.
6. Sprinkle the broccoli with black pepper and toss to combine.

Nutritional Information (per serving):

Calories: 120 Protein: 4g Sodium: 150mg Fiber: 2g Potassium:

120mg Phosphorus: 60mg Carbohydrates: 16g

Mushroom and Spinach Risotto:

Prep Time: 15 minutes Cook Time: 30 minutes Servings: 4

Ingredients:

- 1 cup Arborio rice
- 1 lb (450 g) fresh mushrooms, sliced
- 1 medium onion, finely chopped
- 2 cloves garlic, minced
- 4 cups low-sodium vegetable broth
- 1 cup fresh spinach, chopped
- 1/4 cup grated Parmesan cheese
- 2 tbsps olive oil
- A pinch of Salt(if required)/ salt-free spice
- Pepper to taste
- Fresh parsley for garnish

Directions:

1. Heat the olive oil in a big saucepan over medium heat. Add the minced garlic and diced onion. Sauté until the onion is translucent.
2. Add the sliced mushrooms and sauté them until they give off moisture and begin to turn brown.
3. Stir in the Arborio rice and cook for a couple of minutes until it's lightly toasted.
4. Stir continuously as you gradually add the vegetable broth, one ladleful at a time. Let it soak before adding extra liquid.
5. Keep adding broth and stirring until the rice is cooked through and creamy, in about 20-25 minutes. Adjust the seasoning with salt(optional) and pepper.
6. Stir in the grated Parmesan cheese and chopped spinach. Cook for a further 2-3 minutes, just until the spinach wilts.
7. Take off the heat and allow it to rest for a few minutes.

8. Serve the mushroom and spinach risotto hot, garnished with fresh parsley.

Nutritional Information (per serving):

Calories: 280 kcal Protein: 8g Sodium: 250mg Fiber: 3g Potassium: 300mg Phosphorus: 150mg Carbohydrates: 50g

Minestrone Soup

Prep Time: 15 minutes Cook Time: 30 minutes Servings: 6

Ingredients:

- 1 tbsp olive oil
- 1 medium onion, diced
- 2 cloves garlic, minced
- 2 carrots, shredded
- 2 celery stalks, chopped
- 1 medium zucchini, diced
- 1 cup green beans (canned, no salt added), rinsed & drained
- 1 (14 oz) can diced tomatoes (no salt added)
- 4 cups low-sodium chicken broth
- 1 tsp each: dried basil, dried oregano, black pepper
- 1 ½ cups elbow macaroni
- Fresh basil sprig (garnish)

Directions:

1. In a big saucepan or Dutch oven, warm the olive oil over medium heat. Add and cook the chopped onion for two to three minutes or until it becomes translucent.
2. Toss in the diced zucchini, shredded carrot, chopped celery, and minced garlic. Add the fresh green beans now if using them. Cook until the veggies are tender, about 5 minutes.
3. Stir in the ground black pepper, dried oregano, dry basil, and canned green beans.

4. Pour in the diced tomatoes (plus the juice!) and the low-sodium chicken broth. Bring the mixture to a boil. Lower the heat to a simmer, and let simmer for 10 minutes.
5. Add the dry elbow macaroni to the pot and cook according to the package directions, about 8-10 minutes or until the macaroni is tender.
6. Garnish with a sprig of fresh basil.
7. Ladle the hot minestrone soup into bowls and enjoy!

Nutritional Information (per serving):

Calories: 144 Carbohydrates: 21.9g Dietary Fiber: 2.8g Protein: 5.9g Sodium: 55.1mg Potassium: 355.2mg Phosphorus: 97.8 mg

Baked Tilapia with Fresh Herbs

Prep Time: 15 mins | Cook Time: 20 mins | Servings: 4

Ingredients:

- 4 tilapia fillets
- 1 tbsp olive oil
- Juice of ½ lemon
- 1 clove garlic, minced
- 1 tbsp each: chopped parsley, chopped basil
- ½ tsp black pepper
- Lemon slices (garnish)

Directions:

1. Set the oven temperature to 375°F (190°C). Use parchment paper to line a baking sheet.
2. Make the herb marinade by thoroughly combining the olive oil, lemon juice, black pepper, parsley, basil, and chopped garlic in a small bowl.

3. Lay the tilapia fillets on the prepared baking sheet. Brush them generously with the marinade, making sure to coat both sides well.
4. Bake in the preheated oven for about 20 minutes or until the fish flakes easily with a fork.
5. Remove from the oven and allow it to rest for a few minutes.
6. Serve the fillet with a lemon slice for extra flavor and garnish.

Nutritional Information (per serving):

Calories: 205 Protein: 34g Sodium: 70mg Fiber: 0.5g Potassium: 380mg Phosphorus: 240mg Carbs: 1g

Pork Tenderloin with Apple Chutney

Prep Time: 20 mins | Cook Time: 30 mins | Servings: 4

Ingredients:

For Pork Tenderloin:

- 1 lb pork tenderloin
- 1 tbsp olive oil
- 1 tsp dried thyme
- ½ tsp black pepper
- ¼ tsp salt (optional) salt-free spice

For Apple Chutney:

- 2 medium apples (low-potassium variety), diced
- ¼ cup chopped celery
- ¼ cup apple cider vinegar
- 1 tbsp honey (or less, to taste)
- ¼ tsp ground cinnamon
- ⅛ tsp ground nutmeg
- A pinch of Salt(if required)/ salt-free spice

Directions:

1. Set the oven temperature to 375°F (190°C).
2. Apply a mixture of olive oil, thyme, black pepper, and salt (if desired) on the pork tenderloin. Put it in a roasting pan.
3. Put into the preheated oven and let it roast for about 25-30 minutes. To make sure it's cooked perfectly, use a meat thermometer and check that the thickest part reads 145°F (63°C). Once it's done, take it out of the oven and let it rest for 5 minutes before slicing.
4. While the pork is roasting, make the apple chutney. Combine the diced apples, chopped celery, apple cider vinegar, honey, cinnamon, nutmeg, and a pinch of salt (if using) in a medium saucepan.
5. Cook the chutney over medium heat, stirring occasionally, until the apples are tender and the mixture has thickened, approximately 15-20 minutes.
6. Slice the rested pork tenderloin and serve it topped with the warm apple chutney.

Nutritional Information (per serving):

Calories: 240 Protein: 24g Sodium: 140mg Fiber: 2g Potassium: 300mg Phosphorus: 200mg Carbs: 15g

Lentil Soup with Spinach

Prep Time: 15 mins | Cook Time: 30 mins | Servings: 4

Ingredients:

- 1 cup red lentils, rinsed
- 1 tbsp olive oil
- 1 small onion, diced

- 2 cloves garlic, minced
- 2 medium carrots, diced
- 2 stalks celery, diced
- 4 cups low-sodium vegetable broth
- 1 tsp dried thyme
- ½ tsp ground black pepper
- 2 cups fresh spinach, chopped
- 1 tbsp lemon juice (optional)

Directions:

1. In a big saucepan over medium heat, heat the olive oil. Add the onion and garlic, and cook for approximately 5 minutes or until the onion becomes translucent.
2. Add the carrots and celery, and continue to cook for an extra 5 minutes, stirring occasionally.
3. Stir in the rinsed lentils, low-sodium vegetable broth, thyme, and black pepper. Bring the mixture to a boil.
4. Lower the heat, cover the pan and let it simmer for around 20 minutes or until the lentils are tender.
5. Toss in the chopped spinach and let it cook for another 5 minutes or until it's wilted and tender.
6. Stir in the lemon juice just before serving, if using.

Nutritional Information (per serving):

Calories: 220 Protein: 14g Sodium: 130mg Fiber: 8g Potassium: 350mg Phosphorus: 180mg Carbs: 30g

Roasted Chicken with Herbs

Prep Time: 15 mins | Cook Time: 45 mins | Servings: 4

Ingredients:

- 1 whole chicken (3-4 lbs), giblets removed
- 1 tbsp olive oil

- 1 tsp each: dried rosemary, dried thyme
- ½ tsp each: dried sage, black pepper
- 1 lemon, cut into wedge
- Fresh parsley

Directions:

1. Preheat the oven to a degree Fahrenheit of 375(190°C). Rinse the chicken and use a paper towel to dry it
2. Rub the chicken all over with olive oil, then season with rosemary, thyme, sage, and black pepper.
3. Stuff lemon wedges inside the chicken's cavity.
4. Transfer the chicken to a roasting pan, breast-side up. Roast for approximately 45 minutes in the preheated oven or until a meat thermometer inserted into the thickest portion of the thigh registers 165°F (74°C).
5. Once done, take the chicken out of the oven and allow it to rest for 10 minutes before slicing.
6. Serve the chicken garnished with fresh parsley and extra lemon wedges if desired.

Nutritional Information (per serving):

Calories: 240 Protein: 27g Sodium: 110mg Fiber: 1g Potassium: 300mg Phosphorus: 220mg Carbs: 1g

Cobb Salad

Prep Time: 30 minutes Cook Time: 0 minutes Servings: 4

Ingredients:

- 2 cups romaine lettuce
- 1 cup watercress
- ½ small tomato, diced
- 2 slices cooked turkey bacon, chopped
- 4 oz sliced roasted turkey

- ¼ cup crumbled blue cheese
- 2 tbsp chopped chives
- 1 boiled egg, chopped

Directions:

1. Toss together the romaine lettuce and watercress in a large bowl to prepare the salad base.
2. Arrange the diced tomato, chopped turkey bacon, sliced roasted turkey, crumbled blue cheese, chopped chives, and boiled egg over the salad greens.
3. Serve immediately as a refreshing and nutritious meal.

Nutritional Information (per serving):

Calories: 122 Carbohydrates: 2g Dietary Fiber: 0.7g Protein: 14.4g

Sodium: 286mg Potassium: 270mg Phosphorus: 162mg

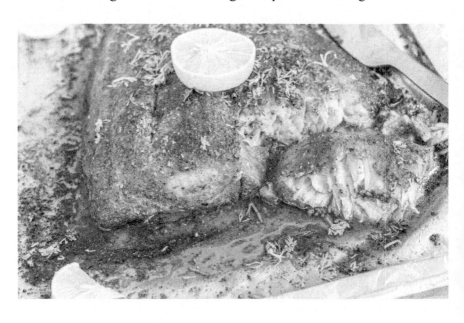

CHAPTER 8

SNACKS RECIPES

Zucchini Sticks

Prep Time: 15 minutes | Cook Time: 20 minutes | Servings: 4

Ingredients:

- 2 medium zucchinis, cut into sticks
- 1/2 cup panko breadcrumbs
- 2 tbsps grated Parmesan cheese
- 1 tbsp dried Italian herbs (such as basil, oregano, or thyme)
- 1/4 tbsp garlic powder
- 1/4 tbsp black pepper
- Cooking spray or olive oil

Directions:

1. Preheat the oven to a Fahrenheit degree of 400 (200°C).
2. Combine the panko breadcrumbs, Parmesan cheese, black pepper, Italian herbs, and garlic powder in a small bowl.
3. Dip each zucchini stick into the breadcrumb mixture and press gently to coat evenly.
4. Line a baking sheet with parchment paper and arrange the coated zucchini sticks on it.
5. Drizzle olive oil over the zucchini sticks or lightly spray with cooking spray.
6. Put it in the oven and bake for 20 minutes or until it's crispy and golden brown.
7. Serve warm with a low-sodium marinara sauce or Greek yogurt dip.

Nutritional Information (per serving):

Calories: 85 Protein: 4g Sodium: 80mg Fiber: 2g Potassium: 195mg Phosphorus: 55mg Carbohydrates: 10g

Apple Cinnamon Chips

Prep Time: 10 mins | Cook Time: 2 hours | Servings: 4

Ingredients:

- 2 large apples (such as Gala or Fuji)
- 1 tbsp ground cinnamon

Directions:

1. Preheat the oven to a temperature of 200°F (93°C). Use parchment paper to line two baking sheets.
2. Cut the apples into very thin slices, approximately 1/8 inch thick.
3. Spread the apple slices in a single layer on the prepared baking sheets.
4. Sprinkle the ground cinnamon evenly over the apple slices.
5. Bake for 1 hour in the preheated oven. Once the apple slices are crisp, turn them over and bake for an extra hour.
6. Allow it to cool fully on the baking sheets before serving.

Nutritional Information (per serving):

Calories: 50 Protein: 2g Sodium: 2mg Fiber: 3g Potassium: 150mg Phosphorus: 10mg Carbs: 14g

Cucumber Sandwiches

Prep Time: 15 mins | Cook Time: 0 mins | Servings: 4

Ingredients:

- 1 large cucumber, thinly sliced

- 4 oz low-sodium cream cheese, softened
- 1 tbsp fresh dill, chopped
- Black pepper to taste
- Optional: low-sodium, high-fiber bread slices (in moderation)

Directions:

1. In a small bowl, thoroughly combine the cream cheese, chopped dill, and a dash of black pepper.
2. Cut the cucumber into extremely thin slices.
3. Apply a thin coating of the cream cheese mixture to half of the cucumber slices for the classic no-bread version. Add a second slice of cucumber on top to create little "sandwiches."
4. For the bread version, spread the cream cheese mixture on a slice of low-sodium, high-fiber bread. Arrange some cucumber slices on top, then cover it with another slice of bread. Cut into desired shapes.
5. Arrange the cucumber sandwiches on a platter and serve immediately.

Nutritional Information (per serving) without bread:

Calories: 60 Protein: 2g Sodium: 65mg Fiber: 1g Potassium: 180mg Phosphorus: 20mg Carbs: 4g

Additional Information: If you are incorporating bread, choose a low-sodium, high-fiber variety to maintain the balance of nutrients. Bread can increase the overall carbohydrate, sodium, and potentially phosphorus content, so it should be consumed in moderation, especially for those managing stage 3 kidney disease.

Roasted Cauliflower and Green Bean Bites

Prep Time: 10 mins | Cook Time: 25 mins | Servings: 4

Ingredients:

- 1/2 large head of cauliflower, cut into bite-sized florets
- 1 cup green beans, trimmed and halved
- 2 tbsps olive oil
- 1 tbsp garlic powder
- 1/2 tbsp paprika
- 1/4 tbsp black pepper
- A pinch of Salt(if required)/ salt-free spice

Directions:

1. Preheat the oven to a temperature of 425°F (220°C). use parchment paper to line a baking sheet.
2. Place the green beans and cauliflower florets in a big basin and mix them with olive oil, paprika, garlic powder, and black pepper until well coated.
3. Arrange the green beans and cauliflower on the prepared baking sheet in a single layer.
4. Roast for 25 minutes in the preheated oven or until the veggies are crisp-tender and golden brown around the edges. To guarantee even cooking, stir halfway through.
5. Take it out from the oven and allow it to cool a bit before serving.

Nutritional Information (per serving):

Calories: 90 Protein: 2g Sodium: 30mg (if no salt added) Fiber: 2g

Potassium: 150mg Phosphorus: 40mg Carbs: 8g

Crispy Kale Chips

Prep Time: 10 minutes Cook Time: 20 minutes Servings: 4

Ingredients:

- 1 bunch of fresh kale, torn
- 1 tbsp olive oil
- A pinch of Salt(if required)/ salt-free spice
- Pepper to taste
- Optional: nutritional yeast or grated Parmesan cheese

Directions:

1. Set the oven temperature to 175°C or 350°F.
2. Thoroughly wash the kale and cut off any tough stems. Cut the leaves into bite-sized pieces.
3. Combine salt(optional), pepper, and olive oil with the shredded kale in a big bowl. To provide a uniform coating, massage the oil into the leaves.
4. Arrange the kale on a parchment paper-lined baking sheet in a single layer.
5. Bake the kale for 15-20 minutes or until it is crispy and gently browned.
6. Take it out from the oven and let it rest for some minutes before serving.
7. Optional: Sprinkle with nutritional yeast or grated Parmesan cheese for added flavor.

Nutritional Information (per serving):

Calories: 60   Protein: 2g   Sodium: 100mg   Fiber: 2g

Potassium: 200mg Phosphorus: 40mg Carbohydrates: 8g

Baked Apple Wedges

Prep Time: 10 mins | Cook Time: 20 mins | Servings: 4

Ingredients:

- 4 medium apples (Gala or Fuji)
- 1 tbsp ground cinnamon
- ¼ tbsp ground nutmeg
- Optional: sprinkle of honey or sugar substitute

Directions:

1. Set the oven temperature to 190°C or 375°F. Use parchment paper to line a baking sheet
2. Core the apples and cut them into wedges, about 8 wedges per apple.
3. Combine the nutmeg and ground cinnamon with the apple wedges in a large bowl. Sprinkle with a sugar substitute or lightly drizzle with honey, if preferred.
4. Spread out the apple wedges on the prepared baking sheet in a single layer.
5. Bake for 20 minutes in the preheated oven or until the apples are tender and slightly caramelized. Flip the wedges over halfway through
6. Take out the wedges from the oven and let it cool a bit before serving.

Nutritional Information (per serving):

Calories: 95 Protein: 0g Sodium: 0mg Fiber: 3g Potassium: 150mg

Phosphorus: 10mg Carbs: 25g

Coleslaw

Prep Time: 15 mins | Cook Time: 0 mins | Servings: 4

Ingredients:

- 2 cups shredded green cabbage
- 1 cup shredded red cabbage
- 1 medium carrot, shredded
- ¼ cup low-fat plain Greek yogurt
- 1 tbsp apple cider vinegar
- 1 tbsp honey or sugar substitute
- ¼ tsp black pepper
- A pinch of Salt(if required)/ salt-free spice

Directions:

1. Combine the carrot, red cabbage, and green cabbage shreds in a big bowl.
2. Combine the Greek yogurt, apple cider vinegar, black pepper, and honey (or sugar replacement) in another small dish. Omit the salt or use a very small amount to keep the sodium low.
3. Pour the dressing over the carrot and cabbage blend and toss well for an even coating.
4. Allow the coleslaw sit for around 10 minutes to allow the flavors to meld before serving.

Nutritional Information (per serving):

Calories: 60 Protein: 2g Sodium: 25mg (if no salt added) Fiber: 2g

Potassium: 180mg Phosphorus: 30mg Carbs: 12g

Flour Tortilla Chips

Prep Time: 10 mins | Cook Time: 10 mins | Servings: 4

Ingredients:

- 4 small low-sodium flour tortillas (whole wheat preferred)
- 1 tbsp olive oil
- ½ tsp paprika
- ¼ tsp garlic powder
- A pinch of Salt(if required)/ salt-free spice

Directions:

1. Set the oven temperature to 175°C or 350°F. Use parchment paper to line a baking sheet
2. Brush each tortilla with olive oil. Then, sprinkle paprika and garlic powder evenly over the tortillas. If using, add a very small pinch of salt or use salt-free spices.
3. Cut the tortillas into triangles or desired shapes using a pizza cutter or sharp knife.
4. Place the tortilla pieces on the prepared baking sheet in a single layer.
5. Bake for a total of 10 minutes in a preheated oven or until the chips are golden brown and crispy. For uniform baking, flip the chips halfway through.
6. Take out from the oven and allow for a few minutes to cool on the baking sheet before serving.

Nutritional Information (per serving):

Calories: 120 Protein: 3g Sodium: 60mg (if no salt added) Fiber: 2g

Potassium: 100mg Phosphorus: 50mg Carbs: 18g

Carrot and Celery Sticks

Prep Time: 10 minutes Cook Time: 0 Servings: 4

Ingredients:

- 4 large carrots, cut into sticks
- 4 celery stalks, cut into sticks
- Hummus or Greek yogurt dip (optional)

Directions:

1. Wash and peel the carrots. Cut them into sticks about 3-4 inches long.
2. Wash the celery stalks and cut them into similar-sized sticks.
3. Place the carrot and celery sticks on a serving platter.
4. Serve with a side of hummus or Greek yogurt dip for added flavor and protein.

Nutritional Information (per serving):

Calories: 30 Protein: 1g Sodium: 60mg Fiber: 2g Potassium: 200mg

Phosphorus: 20mg Carbohydrates: 7g

Pineapple Bar Cookies

Prep Time: 15 mins | Cook Time: 25 mins | Servings: 4

Ingredients:

- 1 cup all-purpose flour
- 1/4 tbsp baking soda
- 1/4 cup unsalted butter, softened
- 1/3 cup sugar or a sugar substitute
- 1 egg
- 1/2 cup crushed pineapple, drained well
- 1 tbsp vanilla extract

Directions:

1. Set the oven to 175°C or350°F Then using parchment paper to line an 8x8 inch baking pan
2. Combine the flour and baking soda in a small basin.
3. Cream together the butter and sugar in a bigger basin until it turns light and fluffy. Add the egg and vanilla extract and mix thoroughly.
4. Pour in crushed pineapple into the wet ingredients.
5. Gradually add the flour and baking soda to the wet mixture, stirring until everything is well combined.
6. Spread the batter evenly into the prepared baking pan.
7. Bake in the oven for 25 minutes, or until a toothpick inserted into the middle comes out clean, and the sides are golden brown.
8. Remove from heat and allow to cool in the pan before cutting them into bars.
9. Serve and enjoy.

Nutritional Information (per serving):

Calories: 210 Protein: 3g Sodium: 45mg Fiber: 1g Potassium: 80mg

Phosphorus: 60mg Carbs: 30g

Granola Bars

Prep Time: 15 mins | Cook Time: 20 mins | Servings: 4

Ingredients:

- 1 cup rolled oats (or less if watching phosphorus)
- 2 tbsp pumpkin seeds
- ¼ cup dried cranberries
- 2 tbsp honey (or substitute)
- 1 tbsp melted unsalted butter
- ½ tsp vanilla extract
- A pinch of Salt(if required)/ salt-free spice

Directions:

1. Set your oven to 163°C or 325°F. Use parchment paper to line an 8x8-inch baking pan.
2. In a large bowl, combine the rolled oats, pumpkin seeds, and dried cranberries.
3. In another small bowl, combine the honey, melted butter, and vanilla extract. If desired, add a very small pinch of salt(optional) or salt-free spice.
4. Pour the wet ingredients over the dry ingredients and mix everything together until it's all well coated
5. Press the mixture firmly into the prepared baking pan.
6. Bake in the preheated oven for 20 minutes or until the edges are golden brown.
7. Allow the granola bars to cool fully in the pan before cutting them into bars
8. Serve and enjoy.

Nutritional Information (per serving):

Calories: 160 Protein: 3g Sodium: 15mg Fiber: 2g Potassium: 140mg Phosphorus: 60mg Carbs: 20g

Low-Sodium Flour Tortilla Chips

Prep Time: 5 minutes Cook Time: 10 minutes Servings: 4

Ingredients:

- 4 large whole wheat/low-sodium tortillas
- 1 tbsp olive oil
- A pinch of Salt(if required)/ salt-free spice

Directions:

1. Set the oven temperature to 175°C or 350°F.
2. Apply olive oil to each tortilla's two sides.

3. Pile the tortillas atop each other and cut them into wedges (like pizza slices).
4. Spread out the tortilla wedges on a baking sheet covered with parchment paper in a single layer.
5. If desired, sprinkle a pinch of salt(optional) over the wedges
6. Bake the chips for 8 to 10 minutes or until they are crispy and golden brown.
7. Allow them to cool slightly before serving.

Nutritional Information (per serving):

Calories: 120 Protein: 2g Sodium: 50mg Fiber: 1g Potassium: 50mg

Phosphorus: 40mg Carbohydrates: 20g

Pear & Almond Parfait

Prep Time: 10 mins | Cook Time: 0 mins | Servings: 4

Ingredients:

- 2 medium pears, cored & diced
- 1 cup low-fat Greek yogurt
- ¼ cup slivered almonds (or less)
- 2 tbsp honey (or substitute)
- ½ tsp ground cinnamon

Directions:

1. Place the Greek yogurt in a small dish and mix it well with ground cinnamon and honey (or sugar replacement).
2. Take four serving glasses or bowls. Layer the bottom of each with a portion of the diced pears.
3. Spoon a layer of the sweetened Greek yogurt over the pears in each glass.
4. Top the yogurt with a sprinkling of slivered almonds.
5. Continue layering until all the ingredients are used, and then top with almonds as garnish.

Nutritional Information (per serving):

Calories: 150 Protein: 6g Sodium: 30mg Fiber: 3g Potassium: 180mg Phosphorus: 80mg Carbs: 22g

Apple Caramel Crisp

Prep Time: 15 mins | Cook Time: 30 mins | Servings: 4

Ingredients:

- 1-2 medium apples (Gala or Fuji), peeled, cored, and sliced
- 2 tbsp caramel
- ¼ cup rolled oats
- 2 tbsp all-purpose flour
- 2 tbsp brown sugar (or sugar substitute)
- 2 tbsps unsalted butter, cubed
- ¼ tbsp ground cinnamon

Directions:

1. Set the oven to 175°C, or 350°F. Grease a smaller baking dish very lightly.
2. Line the bottom of the prepared dish with the apple slices. Evenly drizzle the apples with the caramel sauce.
3. Thoroughly combine the flour, cinnamon, brown sugar (or sugar substitute), and rolled oats in a bowl.
4. Add the unsalted butter cubes to the oat mixture. Using your fingertips or a fork, mix in the butter until the mixture looks like coarse crumbs.
5. Evenly sprinkle the crumb topping over the apples with caramel coating.
6. Bake in the preheated for 30 minutes, or until the apples are soft and the topping is golden brown.
7. Let it cool for a few minutes before serving.

Nutritional Information (per serving):

Calories: 180 Protein: 1g Sodium: 15mg Fiber: 2g Potassium: 120mg Phosphorus: 40mg Carbs: 30g

Baked Tofu Cubes

Prep Time: 15 minutes Cook Time: 30 minutes Servings: 4

Ingredients:

- 1 block extra-firm tofu (14 oz)
- 1 tbsp low-sodium soy sauce
- 1 tbsp olive oil
- 1 tsp each: garlic powder, onion powder
- ½ tsp each: black pepper, dried thyme (optional)

Directions:

1. Set the oven to a temperature of 375°F or 190°C.
2. Press and drain the tofu to get rid of extra water. Cut it into 1-inch cubes.
3. Combine the soy sauce, olive oil, onion and garlic powders, black pepper, and dried thyme (if using) in a bowl.
4. Pour the tofu cubes into the bowl and toss just enough to coat with the marinade.
5. Place the tofu cubes on a parchment-lined baking sheet.
6. Bake the cubes for 30 minutes, flipping them halfway through or until they are crispy and golden.
7. Serve warm as a snack or add them to salads, stir-fries, or grain bowls.

Nutritional Information (per serving):

Calories: 120 Protein: 12g Sodium: 150mg Fiber: 2g Potassium: 180mg Phosphorus: 100mg Carbohydrates: 5g

CHAPTER 9

DESSERTS RECIPES

Caramel-Coated Pretzels

Prep Time: 10 minutes Cook Time: 20 minutes Servings: 8

Ingredients:

- 1 cup unsalted pretzels
- ½ cup granulated sugar
- ¼ cup unsalted butter
- ¼ cup low-potassium corn syrup
- ¼ tsp salt (optional)
- Cooking spray

Directions:

1. Set your oven to a temperature of 350°F (175°C).
2. Use parchment paper to line a baking sheet and then grease lightly grease with cooking spray.
3. Spread out the pretzels on the baking sheet in a single layer.
4. Put the butter, corn syrup, and sugar in a saucepan. Stir the mixture while heating over medium-low heat until it becomes smooth and the sugar dissolves.
5. Bring the mixture to a gentle boil, then turn off the heat.
6. Gently drizzle the caramel blend over the pretzels, ensuring they are evenly coated.
7. Bake the pretzels for 10 minutes in the preheated oven, flipping them halfway through
8. Take out the pretzels from the oven and allow for complete cooling on the baking sheet.
9. Once cooled, break apart any clusters of pretzels. Serve and enjoy.

Nutritional Information (per serving):

Calories: 120 Protein: 1g Sodium: 50mg Fiber: 0g Potassium: 20mg Phosphorus: 10mg Carbohydrates: 27g

Berry Fruit Salad

Prep Time: 10 mins | Cook Time: 0 mins | Servings: 4

Ingredients:

- 1 cup strawberries, halved
- 1 cup blueberries
- 1 cup blackberries
- 1 cup raspberries
- 2 tbsps honey or a sugar substitute
- 1 tbsp lemon juice (optional)

Directions:

1. Combine the raspberries, blackberries, blueberries, and strawberries in a big basin.
2. Drizzle the berries with honey or a sugar substitute. If using, add the lemon juice.
3. Gently mix the berries in the lemon juice and honey until well coated.
4. Let the salad sit for about 5 minutes to allow the flavors to meld before serving.

Nutritional Information (per serving):

Calories: 70 Protein: 1g Sodium: 0mg Fiber: 5g Potassium: 150mg Phosphorus: 35mg Carbs: 17g

Marshmallow Popcorn Balls

Prep Time: 15 minutes Cook Time: 10 minutes Servings: 10

Ingredients:

- 8 cups air-popped popcorn (unsalted)
- 1 cup mini marshmallows (low-sodium)
- 2 tbsp unsalted butter
- ¼ tsp vanilla extract
- Cooking spray

Directions:

1. Put the air-popped popcorn in a large mixing dish.
2. Melt the butter in a saucepan over low heat.
3. Add the mini marshmallows to the melted butter and stir until smooth.
4. Take the saucepan off the heat and stir in the vanilla extract.
5. Pour the marshmallow mixture over the popcorn and gently toss to coat evenly.
6. Roll the coated popcorn into balls by rubbing your hands with cooking spray to keep them from sticking.
7. Place the popcorn balls on a parchment-lined tray to set.
8. Let them cool fully before serving.

Nutritional Information (per serving):

Calories: 120 Protein: 1g Sodium: 10mg Fiber: 1g Potassium: 20mg

Phosphorus: 10mg Carbohydrates: 27g

Blueberry Crumble

Prep Time: 15 minutes Cook Time: 30 minutes Servings: 6

Ingredients:

- 3 cups fresh blueberries
- 1 tbsp lemon juice
- ¼ cup granulated sugar
- ½ cup all-purpose flour
- ¼ cup rolled oats
- 2 tbsps unsalted butter
- ¼ tbsp cinnamon
- Cooking spray

Directions:

1. Set the oven temperature to 175°C or 350°F.
2. Put the blueberries, half of the granulated sugar, and lemon juice in a mixing dish. Coat the blueberries by gently tossing them.
3. Combine the flour, oats, cinnamon, and remaining sugar in another bowl.
4. Add the butter, cut into tiny pieces, to the flour mixture. Crumble the butter into the dry ingredients using your fingers.
5. Grease a baking dish with cooking spray and spread the blueberry blend evenly.
6. Scatter the crumble topping atop the blueberries.
7. Bake for 25-30 minutes in the preheated oven or until the topping is golden brown and the blueberries are bubbling.
8. Allow it to cool a little before serving.

Nutritional Information (per serving):

Calories: 150 Protein: 2g Sodium: 5mg Fiber: 3g Potassium: 50mg

Phosphorus: 30mg Carbohydrates: 30g

Strawberry Sorbet

Prep Time: 15 mins | Cook Time: 0 mins | Servings: 4

Ingredients:

- 2 cups fresh strawberries, hulled
- ¼ cup sugar (or substitute)
- 1 tbsp lemon juice

Directions:

1. Puree the strawberries in a food processor or blender until they are smooth.
2. Mix the strawberry puree with the sugar (or sugar alternative) and lemon juice. Blend further until all the ingredients are thoroughly combined.
3. Pour the mixture into a shallow dish and place it in the freezer.
4. Use a fork to stir the mixture every 30 minutes to break up any ice crystals until the sorbet is smooth and evenly frozen, which should take two to three hours.
5. To serve the sorbet with a softer texture, serve it right away; to serve it with a harder consistency, freeze it solid and let it thaw for a few minutes.

Nutritional Information (per serving):

Calories: 50 Protein: 0g Sodium: 0mg Fiber: 2g Potassium: 110mg

Phosphorus: 15mg Carbs: 13g

Berry Beet Smoothie Bowl

Prep Time: 10 minutes Cook Time: 0 minute Servings: 2

Ingredients:

- 1 small cooked beet, peeled
- 1 cup mixed berries (blueberries, raspberries, and strawberries)
- ½ cup low-potassium yogurt
- 1 tbsp chia seeds
- 1 tbsp honey (optional)
- Fresh mint leaves

Directions:

1. Put the yogurt, chia seeds, mixed berries, and cooked beet into a blender.
2. Blend until creamy and smooth. If necessary, adjust the consistency by adding extra yogurt.
3. Taste and, if desired, sweeten with honey (use moderately).
4. Transfer the smoothie mixture to bowls.
5. Add some mint leaves as a garnish.
6. Serve immediately and enjoy!

Nutritional Information (per serving):

Calories: 120 Protein: 4g Sodium: 20mg Fiber: 5g Potassium: 150mg Phosphorus: 60mg Carbohydrates: 20g

Pumpkin Custard

Prep Time: 10 mins | Cook Time: 30 mins | Servings: 4

Ingredients:

- 1 cup pumpkin puree (not pie filling)
- 1 cup low-fat milk
- 2 eggs
- ¼ cup sugar (or substitute)
- 1 tsp vanilla extract
- ½ tsp ground cinnamon
- ¼ tsp each: ground nutmeg, ground ginger

Directions:

1. Set the oven temperature to 175°C, or 350°F. Grease a small baking dish or four ramekins.
2. Put the eggs, low-fat milk, sugar (or sugar substitute), vanilla extract, cinnamon, nutmeg, and ginger into a mixing bowl along with the pumpkin puree. Whisk until well combined and smooth.
3. Pour the pumpkin blend into the prepared ramekins or baking dish.
4. Place the ramekins or baking dish in a larger baking pan and fill the pan with hot water halfway up the sides of the ramekins or dish (bain-marie method).
5. Bake for 30 minutes in the preheated oven, or until the custard is set and a knife inserted close to the middle comes out clean.
6. Remove from the oven and allow it to cool a little bit. Serve warm or chill in the refrigerator before serving.

Nutritional Information (per serving):

Calories: 120 Protein: 4g Sodium: 60mg Fiber: 2g Potassium: 180mg Phosphorus: 90mg Carbs: 18g

Almond Biscotti

Prep Time: 20 mins | Cook Time: 40 mins | Servings: 4

Ingredients:

- 1 cup almond flour
- ¼ cup sugar (or substitute)
- 1 egg
- ½ tsp vanilla extract
- ¼ tsp low-sodium baking powder
- ¼ cup slivered almonds

Directions:

1. Set the oven temperature to 325°F or 165°C. Use parchment paper to line a baking sheet.
2. Combine the almond flour, sugar (or sugar substitute), and baking powder in a large basin.
3. Beat the egg and vanilla extract together thoroughly in another basin.
4. Combine the wet and dry ingredients and stir until a dough forms. Stir in the almond slices.
5. Shape the dough into a log approximately 2 inches wide and place it on the prepared baking sheet.
6. Bake for 25 minutes in the preheated oven, or until the log is firm to the touch.
7. Take out from heat and allow it to cool for 10 minutes. Cut the log into 1/2-inch-thick slices.
8. Put the slices back on the baking sheet, cut side down, and bake for an extra 15 minutes, or until the biscotti are golden and crisp.
9. Allow it to cool fully on a wire rack before serving.

Nutritional Information (per serving):

Calories: 200 Protein: 6g Sodium: 30mg Fiber: 3g Potassium: 100mg Phosphorus: 80mg Carbs: 10g

Blueberry Muffins

Prep Time: 10 mins | Cook Time: 20 mins | Servings: 4

Ingredients:

- 1 cup whole wheat flour
- ½ cup fresh blueberries
- ¼ cup sugar (or substitute)
- ½ cup low-fat milk

- 1 egg
- 1 tbsp vanilla extract
- 1 tbsp low-sodium baking powder
- ¼ cup melted unsalted butter

Directions:

1. Set the oven temperature to 375°F or 190°C. Use paper liners or unsalted butter to grease or line a muffin pan.
2. Combine the baking powder, sugar (or sugar substitute), and whole wheat flour in a bowl.
3. Combine the melted butter, low-fat milk, egg, and vanilla extract in a separate dish.
4. Gently stir the dry and wet ingredients until well combined. Add the blueberries and fold gently.
5. Evenly divide the batter between the muffin cups.
6. Bake for 20 minutes, or until a toothpick put into a muffin comes out clean.
7. Let cool before serving.

Nutritional Information (per serving):

Calories: 180 Protein: 4g Sodium: 55mg Fiber: 2g Potassium: 90mg Phosphorus: 70mg Carbs: 30g

Carrot Cake Squares

Prep Time: 15 mins | Cook Time: 25 mins | Servings: 4

Ingredients:

- 1 cup whole wheat flour
- ½ cup grated carrots
- ¼ cup unsweetened applesauce
- ¼ cup sugar (or substitute)
- 1 egg
- 1 tbsp vanilla extract

- ½ tbsp low-sodium baking soda
- ½ tbsp ground cinnamon
- ¼ tbsp ground nutmeg

Directions:

1. Set the oven temperature to 175°C or 350°F. Use parchment paper to line an 8x 8-inch baking pan
2. Mix the nutmeg, cinnamon, baking soda, and whole wheat flour in a large basin.
3. Combine the applesauce, egg, vanilla extract, sugar (or sugar substitute), and shredded carrots in another bowl.
4. Gently stir the dry and wet ingredients until well combined.
5. Evenly distribute the batter into the prepared pan.
6. Bake for 25 minutes in the preheated oven, or until a toothpick injected into the center comes out clean.
7. Allow to cool before cutting into squares and serving.

Nutritional Information (per serving):

Calories: 150 Protein: 3g Sodium: 50mg Fiber: 3g Potassium: 120mg Phosphorus: 60mg Carbs: 28g

Tapioca Pudding

Prep Time: 10 mins | Cook Time: 15 mins | Servings: 4

Ingredients:

- ¼ cup small pearl tapioca
- 1 ½ cups low-fat milk
- ¼ cup sugar (or substitute)
- 1 egg, beaten
- 1 tsp vanilla extract

Directions:

1. Soak the tapioca pearls in water for 30 minutes, then drain.

2. Put the soaked tapioca, low-fat milk, and sugar (or sugar replacement) in a saucepan. Stirring regularly, cook over medium heat until mixture reaches a simmer.
3. Lower the heat to low and simmer, stirring regularly, until the pudding thickens and the tapioca pearls become translucent, about 10 to 15 minutes.
4. To temper the beaten egg, softly whisk a tiny bit of the heated mixture into it. Then, gradually stir the egg back into the pudding.
5. Cook for an extra 2 minutes, stirring constantly, to ensure the egg is fully cooked.
6. Turn off the heat and whisk in the vanilla extract.
7. Transfer the pudding to serving plates and let it cool to room temperature. Refrigerate it to chill before serving.

Nutritional Information (per serving):

Calories: 140 Protein: 4g Sodium: 45mg Fiber: 0g Potassium: 120mg Phosphorus: 80mg Carbs: 25g

Rice Cereal Treats

Prep Time: 30 minutes Cook Time: 1 hour Servings: 9 squares

Ingredients:

- 1 ½ cups mini marshmallows
- ¼ cup sugar substitute
- 3 cups rice cereal
- 1 tbsp butter or margarine

Directions:

1. In a large saucepan, melt the butter or margarine over low heat.
2. Add the marshmallows and stir constantly until they melt.
3. Stir in your chosen sugar alternative.

4. Add the rice cereal and stir until well combined.
5. Transfer the mixture into a greased 8 x 8 pan.
6. Apply wax paper to press it down.
7. Allow it to cool, and then cut it into nine squares.

Nutritional Information (per square):

Calories: 77 Carbs: 16g Fiber: 0.1g Protein: 0.5g Sodium: 11mg
Potassium: 5mg Phosphorus: 6mg

Cranberry–Raspberry Gelatin Salad

Prep Time: 30 minutes Cook Time: 2 hours Servings: 1 cup per serving

Ingredients:

- 1 can whole cranberry sauce
- 1 box (0.3 oz) raspberry gelatin
- 1 cup ginger ale
- 1 cup frozen raspberries
- ½ cup chopped celery

Directions:

1. Boil 1 cup water for gelatin. Mix with 1 can of cranberry sauce and pour into a large glass serving bowl.
2. Add 1 cup of ginger ale, 1 cup of frozen raspberries, and ½ cup of chopped celery.
3. Chill in the refrigerator for two hours or until solid.
4. Serve and enjoy

Nutritional Information (per serving):

Calories: 59 kcal Protein: 0.6 g Sodium: 21mg Fiber: 1g Potassium: 45mg Phosphorus: 7mg Carbs: 14.3g

Blueberry Lemon Pound Cake

Prep Time: 15 minutes Cook Time: 1 hour Servings: 10 slices

Ingredients:

- 1 cup fresh blueberries
- 1 ½ cups all-purpose flour
- 1 tsp baking powder
- ½ tsp baking soda
- ¼ tsp salt(optional) or salt-free spices
- ½ cup unsalted butter, softened
- ¾ cup granulated sugar
- 2 large eggs
- Zest of 1 lemon
- Juice of 1 lemon
- ½ cup low-fat milk

Directions:

1. Set the oven temperature to 175°C or 350°F. Grease and flour a loaf pan
2. Combine the flour, baking soda, baking powder, and salt(optional) in a medium-sized bowl.
3. Cream the sugar and softened butter together in a different, big basin until they are light and fluffy.
4. Beat in the eggs, one at a time, followed by the lemon zest and juice.
5. Gradually add the dry ingredients to the wet ingredients, alternating with the milk. Mix until just combined.
6. Gently fold in the fresh blueberries.
7. Pour the batter into the prepared loaf pan.
8. Bake for 50-60 minutes or until a toothpick injected into the center comes out clean.
9. Let the cake cool in the pan for 10 minutes, then transfer to a wire rack to cool completely.

Nutritional Information (per slice):

Calories: 180   Protein: 3g   Sodium: 80mg   Fiber: 1g

Potassium: 100mg Phosphorus: 60mg Carbs: 25g

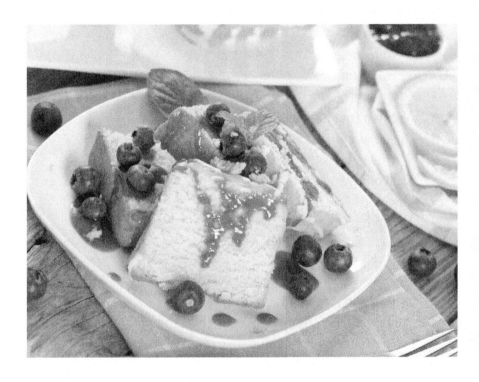

CHAPTER 10

BEVERAGES

Raspberry-Lime Water

Prep Time: 5 minutes Servings: 2

Ingredients:

- 1 cup fresh raspberries
- Juice of 2 limes
- 4 cups cold water
- Ice cubes (optional)
- Fresh mint leaves (garnish)

Directions:

1. Wash the raspberries thoroughly with cold water.
2. Put together the lime juice and raspberries in a pitcher.
3. Gently muddle the raspberries with a spoon or muddler to release their flavor.
4. Pour in cold water and thoroughly mix.
5. Refrigerate for a minimum of 1 hour to allow the flavors to meld.
6. Garnish with fresh mint leaves and serve cold over ice cubes.

Nutritional Information (per serving):

Calories: 15 Protein: 0.5g Sodium: 0mg Fiber: 4g Potassium: 60mg

Phosphorus: 10mg Carbohydrates: 4g

Nonalcoholic Margarita

Prep Time: 10 minutes Servings: 2

Ingredients:

- 1 cup fresh lime juice
- 1 cup unsweetened orange juice
- 1 tbsp honey or agave syrup
- Ice cubes
- Lime wedges
- Salt (optional, for rimming)

Directions:

1. Combine together the lime juice, orange juice, and honey/agave syrup in a pitcher.
2. Stir thoroughly until the sweetener is melted.
3. If preferred, rim the serving glasses with salt.
4. Fill the glasses with ice cubes.
5. Pour the margarita mixture over the ice.
6. Add lime wedges as a garnish.
7. Serve the margarita chilled.

Nutritional Information (per serving):

Calories: 60 Protein: 0.5g Sodium: 5mg Fiber: 0.5g Potassium: 100mg Phosphorus: 10mg Carbs: 15g

Minty-Lime Iced Tea

Prep Time: 10 minutes (plus chilling time) Cook Time: 5 minutes Servings: 4

Ingredients:

- 4 cups water
- 4 black tea bags

- Juice of 2 limes
- Fresh mint leaves (about ½ cup)
- Ice cubes
- Lime slices (for garnish)

Directions:

1. Heat 4 cups of water till it boils.
2. Take off the heat and put the tea bags in. Soak for five minutes.
3. Take out the tea bags and allow them to cool to room temperature.
4. Squeeze in the lime juice and fresh mint leaves into the cooled tea.
5. Refrigerate for a minimum of 1 hour to allow the flavors to meld.
6. Serve over ice cubes, garnished with lime slices and additional mint leaves.

Nutritional Information (per serving):

Calories: 10 Protein: 0g Sodium: 5mg Fiber: 0g Potassium: 20mg

Phosphorus: 5mg Carbs: 3g

Herbal Iced Tea

Prep Time: 5 mins (plus chilling) | Cook Time: 5 mins | Servings: 4

Ingredients:

- 4 cups water
- 4 herbal tea bags (such as chamomile or peppermint)

Directions:

1. Boil the water and pour over the herbal tea bags in a large pitcher.
2. Let steep for 5 minutes, then remove the tea bags.

3. Allow the tea to cool to room temperature, then refrigerate until chilled.
4. Serve the herbal iced tea over ice.

Nutritional Information (per serving):

Calories: 0 Protein: 0g Sodium: 0mg Fiber: 0g Potassium: 10mg Phosphorus: 0mg Carbs: 0g

Minty-Lime Iced Tea

Prep Time: 10 minutes (plus chilling time) Cook Time: 5 minutes Servings: 4

Ingredients:

- 4 cups water
- 4 black tea bags
- Juice of 2 limes
- Fresh mint leaves (about ½ cup)
- Ice cubes
- Lime slices (for garnish)

Directions:

1. Bring 4 cups of water to a boil.
2. Remove from heat and add the tea bags. Steep for 5 minutes.
3. Remove the tea bags and let the tea cool to room temperature.
4. Add the lime juice and fresh mint leaves to the cooled tea.
5. Chill in the freezer for a minimum of 1 hour to allow the flavors to meld.
6. Top with more mint leaves and lime slices, and serve over ice cubes for garnish.

Nutritional Information (per serving):

Calories: 10 Protein: 0g Sodium: 5mg Fiber: 0g Potassium: 20mg
Phosphorus: 5mg Carbs: 3g

Watermelon-Rosemary Water

Prep Time: 10 minutes Servings: 4

Ingredients:

- 4 cups cubed watermelon (seedless)
- 2 sprigs fresh rosemary
- 4 cups cold water
- Ice cubes
- Watermelon wedges (for garnish)

Directions:

1. Combine together the cubed watermelon and rosemary sprigs in a pitcher.
2. Muddle the watermelon with a muddler to allow the release of its juices.
3. Add the cold water and thoroughly stir.
4. Chill in the refrigerator for a minimum of 1 hour to infuse the flavors.
5. Serve chilled over ice cubes, garnishing each glass with watermelon wedges for a touch of sweetness.

Nutritional Information (per serving):

Calories: 20   Protein: 0.5g   Sodium: 0mg   Fiber: 0.5g
Potassium: 80mg Phosphorus: 10mg Carbohydrates: 5g

Strawberry-Basil Water

Prep Time: 5 minutes Servings: 2

Ingredients:

- 1 cup sliced strawberries
- 6-8 fresh basil leaves
- 2 cups cold water
- Ice cubes

Directions:

1. Combine together the sliced strawberries and basil leaves in a pitcher.
2. Top with the cold water and stir moderately.
3. Chill in the refrigerator for 30 minutes to allow the flavors combine well.
4. Serve chilled over ice cubes.

Nutritional Information (per serving):

Calories: 10 Protein: 0.5g Sodium: 0mg Fiber: 1gbPotassium: 60mg

Phosphorus: 10mg Carbs: 2g

Mint-Lemon Water

Prep Time: 5 minutes Servings: 2

Ingredients:

- Juice of 2 lemons
- 10-12 fresh mint leaves
- 2 cups cold water
- Ice cubes
- Lemon slices (for garnish)

Directions:

1. Combine together the lemon juice and mint leaves in a pitcher.
2. Top with the cold water and stir thoroughly.
3. Chill in the refrigerator for 30 minutes to infuse the flavors.

4. Serve chilled over ice cubes, garnishing each glass with lemon slices.

Nutritional Information (per serving):

Calories: 5 Protein: 0g Sodium: 0mg Fiber: 0g Potassium: 20mg

Phosphorus: 5mg Carbs: 2g

Cranberry Spritzer

Prep Time: 5 minutes Servings: 2

Ingredients:

- 1 cup unsweetened cranberry juice
- 1 cup sparkling water (unsweetened)
- Ice cubes
- Fresh cranberries (for garnish)

Directions:

1. Pour the sparkling water and cranberry juice into a glass.
2. Add ice cubes.
3. Add fresh cranberries as a garnish.
4. Serve immediately.

Nutritional Information (per serving):

Calories: 20 Protein: 0g Sodium: 5mg Fiber: 0g Potassium: 10mg

Phosphorus: 5mg Carbs: 5g

Lemon Lime Soda

Prep Time: 5 mins | Cook Time: 0 mins | Servings: 4

Ingredients:

- 4 cups sparkling water
- Juice of 1 lemon

- Juice of 1 lime
- 1 tbsp sugar substitute (optional)

Directions:

1. Combine together the sparkling water with the freshly squeezed lemon and lime juice in a pitcher.
2. If preferred, add the sugar substitute and stir until it dissolves.
3. Serve chilled or over ice for a fizzy, refreshing drink.

Nutritional Information (per serving):

Calories: 5 Protein: 0g Sodium: 5mg Fiber: 0g Potassium: 20mg

Phosphorus: 0mg Carbs: 2g

Cherry Vanilla Smoothie

Prep Time: 5 mins | Cook Time: 0 mins | Servings: 4

Ingredients:

- 2 cups frozen cherries
- 1 cup low-fat milk or almond milk
- 1 tbsp vanilla extract
- 1 tbsp honey or a sugar substitute

Directions:

1. Put the frozen cherries, almond or low-fat milk, vanilla extract, and honey (or sugar substitute) in a blender.
2. Blend until it achieves a smooth and creamy consistency.
3. Transfer the smoothie into glasses and serve immediately.

Nutritional Information (per serving):

Calories: 80 Protein: 2g Sodium: 30mg Fiber: 2g Potassium: 160mg

Phosphorus: 50mg Carbs: 15g

Green Tea Latte

Prep Time: 5 mins | Cook Time: 5 mins | Servings: 4

Ingredients:

- 4 cups water
- 4 bags decaffeinated green tea
- 2 cups low-fat milk (or almond milk)
- 1 tbsp honey (or substitute)
- ½ tsp vanilla extract (optional)

Directions:

1. Bring the water to a simmer and steep the green tea bags for approximately three minutes. Take out the tea bags.
2. In a small saucepan, heat the low-fat milk or almond milk until it begins to simmer (Avoid boiling.)
3. If desired, add the vanilla extract to the milk and stir.
4. Divide the brewed tea equally among four mugs.
5. Pour in the heated milk over the tea, stirring mildly to combine.
6. Sweeten with honey or a sugar substitute to taste.
7. Serve warm.

Nutritional Information (per serving):

Calories: 60 Protein: 4g Sodium: 40mg Fiber: 0g Potassium: 150mg

Phosphorus: 80mg Carbs: 8g

Blueberry Infused Water

Prep Time: 5 mins | Cook Time: 0 mins | Servings: 4

Ingredients:

- 1 cup fresh blueberries
- 4 cups water

Directions:

1. Put the blueberries in a large pitcher.
2. Add the water and stir mildly.
3. Chill in the refrigerator for a minimum of 2 hours or overnight to allow the flavors to blend.
4. To serve, you can either pour straight into glasses or use a strainer to hold back the blueberries if you prefer.
5. Enjoy.

Nutritional Information (per serving):

Calories: 20 Protein: 0g Sodium: 0mg Fiber: 1g Potassium: 30mg Phosphorus: 5mg Carbs: 5g

Strawberry Smoothie

Prep Time: 5 mins | Cook Time: 0 mins | Servings: 4

Ingredients:

- 2 cups fresh strawberries, hulled
- 1 cup low-fat milk (or almond milk)
- 1 tbsp honey (or substitute)

Directions:

1. Put the strawberries, almond or low-fat milk, and honey (or sugar substitute) in a blender.
2. Blend until it achieves a smooth and creamy consistency.
3. Pour the smoothie into glasses and serve immediately.

Nutritional Information (per serving):

Calories: 60 Protein: 2g Sodium: 30mg Fiber: 2g Potassium: 150mg Phosphorus: 50mg Carbs: 12g

Carrot Ginger Juice

Prep Time: 10 mins | Cook Time: 0 mins | Servings: 4

Ingredients:

- 4 large carrots, peeled
- 1-inch piece of ginger, peeled
- 2 cups water

Directions:

1. Use a juicer to juice the ginger and carrots.
2. Combine the fresh juice and water to dilute the concentration of nutrients, particularly potassium, in the mixture.
3. Serve the juice chilled or over ice.

Nutritional Information (per serving):

Calories: 40 Protein: 1g Sodium: 20mg Fiber: 2g Potassium: 200mg

Phosphorus: 35mg Carbs: 9g

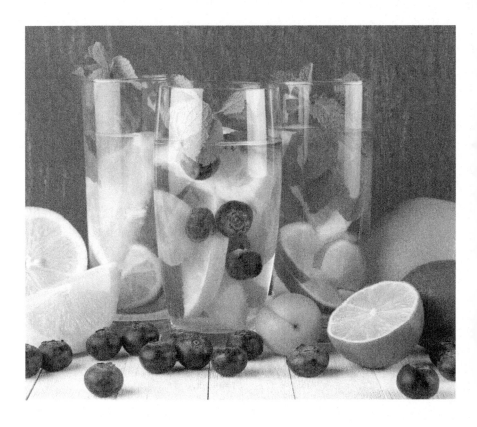

CHAPTER 11

DEBUNKING MYTHS ABOUT KIDNEY DIETS

People who have Stage 3 kidney disease have probably heard a lot of tips on what to eat and what not to eat. Not all the information out there is correct or useful. Some well-meaning advice from family and friends, or even old medical advice, can actually make you feel confused and anxious about the food you choose. The goal of this chapter is to clear up any misperception you may have about kidney diets and give you clarity and confidence.

Myth 1: Kidney-Friendly Food is Bland and Boring

This is absolutely far from being the truth! A kidney-friendly diet does not mean you are stuck with bland and tasteless meals. Rather, it is a perfect opportunity for you to discover a wide range of fresh and flavorful ingredients. There are lots of new herbs and spices to try - rosemary, thyme, cumin, or paprika, which add depth to your food. Also, grilling, roasting, and slow-cooking are ways of cooking that will help to keep your meals healthy and satisfying. You don't have to sacrifice taste!

Myth 2: You Have to Avoid All Fruits and Vegetables

This is another misconception that needs to be trashed. While there's no doubt that some fruits and vegetables have high levels of potassium and, therefore, must be consumed moderately, many fruits and vegetables are very much ideal for a renal diet. Among the great and nutritious foods that are mild on your kidneys are berries, apples, pears, cauliflower, broccoli (in moderation), bell peppers, and cucumbers. A qualified dietician can assist you in designing a food plan with lots of kidney-friendly choices.

Myth 3: All Kidney Diets Are the Same

Completely not! Kidney disease has different stages. Hence, your dietary requirements may vary based on your particular state and health. While some may concentrate more on phosphorous, others might have to monitor their potassium intake strictly. Your doctor and renal dietitian will tailor a diet plan that's specifically designed for your kidneys

Myth 4: You Need to Drink Gallons of Water to "Flush" Your Kidneys

Although it's crucial for everyone to stay hydrated, consuming too much water won't "flush" your kidneys or cure renal disease. In fact, drinking too much water might be dangerous if your kidneys aren't working correctly. Never deviate from your doctor's recommended daily consumption of fluids to avoid straining your kidneys.

Myth 5: You Can't Eat Out If You Have Kidney Disease

Dining out can still be a fun and pleasurable experience with kidney disease! It only involves a little additional planning and conversation with your waiter, but many restaurants provide alternatives that can be adapted to match your diet. Choose foods that are grilled, roasted, or steamed rather than fried. Ask for sauces and dressings on the side so you can control how much you use. Also, don't hesitate to request variations like "no added salt" or exchange high-potassium veggies for lower ones.

Myth 6: Protein is Bad for Your Kidneys

A robust immune system and the growth and maintenance of muscular mass depend on protein. On the other hand, consuming too much protein may overwork your kidneys. For this reason, it's crucial to discuss with your dietician how much protein is appropriate for your particular requirements. They will guide you in selecting lean protein sources and make sure you consume adequately without going overboard.

Myth 7: Once You Start a Kidney Diet, You Can Never Deviate From It

A kidney-friendly diet is a lifestyle change, but it doesn't have to be rigid. With the guidance of your dietitian, you may be able to occasionally enjoy foods that are not typically on your diet. The key is moderation and understanding how to balance your choices over time.

Myth 8: Supplements Can Cure Kidney Disease

While it's tempting to believe that there's a "magic pill" out there that can cure chronic kidney disease (CKD), unfortunately, that's not the case. Supplements may play a helpful role for some people with CKD, but they are not a cure. In fact, taking the wrong supplements without medical guidance can sometimes do more harm than good. Always consult with your doctor or dietitian before adding any supplements to your routine. They'll help determine what's beneficial for you and what to avoid, ensuring your health is protected while you manage your kidney disease. Remember, there's no quick fix, but with the right care, you can manage your condition effectively.

Myth 9: If You Don't Have Symptoms, Your Diet Doesn't Matter

One of the trickiest things about kidney disease is how quietly it can progress, especially in the early stages. Just because you're not experiencing any symptoms doesn't mean everything is fine beneath the surface. That's why your diet plays such an important role, even when you feel perfectly well. By sticking to a kidney-friendly diet, you're helping to protect your kidneys and slow down the progression of the disease. The goal is to preserve your kidney function for as long as possible, so even if you're symptom-free now, your efforts today can make a big difference down the road. It's all about staying one step ahead!

CHAPTER 12

MEDICATIONS, SUPPLEMENTS AND YOUR KIDNEY HEALTH

Overview of Common Medications Used in Kidney Disease

When managing kidney disease, particularly in seniors with stage 3 kidney disease, understanding the medications involved is crucial. These medications are often necessary to control the symptoms and progression of kidney disease, as well as to manage other related health conditions. Here, we will explore some of the most commonly prescribed medications for these patients, with a focus on their purposes and the special considerations needed for kidney health.

1. Antihypertensives (Blood Pressure Medications)

- **ACE Inhibitors (e.g., Lisinopril, Enalapril):** These drugs help relax blood vessels and reduce blood pressure, which can help slow the progression of kidney disease by reducing the pressure on the glomeruli (the kidney's filtering units). However, they need careful monitoring as they can potentially increase potassium levels in the blood and affect kidney function.

- **ARBs (Angiotensin II Receptor Blockers, e.g., Losartan, Valsartan):** Similar to ACE inhibitors, ARBs also help manage high blood pressure and proteinuria (excessive protein in urine), which are common in kidney disease. They are often used as an alternative to ACE inhibitors, especially if cough— a common side effect of ACE inhibitors—becomes problematic.

2. Diuretics

- **Thiazide Diuretics (e.g., Hydrochlorothiazide):** Used to help the body eliminate fluid and sodium through urine, these medications can control blood pressure and help reduce swelling, a common issue in kidney disease. Monitoring of electrolyte levels is necessary as they can lead to decreased potassium levels.

- **Loop Diuretics (e.g., Furosemide):** More potent than thiazide diuretics, loop diuretics are used in cases where there is significant fluid overload, and more aggressive management of fluid retention is needed. They require careful monitoring of kidney function and electrolytes, as they can cause dehydration and mineral imbalances.

3. Medications for Anemia Management

- **Erythropoiesis-Stimulating Agents (ESAs, e.g.,   ):** These drugs are used to stimulate the production of red blood cells, which can be reduced in kidney disease due to the kidneys' reduced ability to produce erythropoietin. While effective, they must be used cautiously to avoid increasing the risk of cardiovascular events.

- **Iron Supplements:** Often administered orally or intravenously in kidney disease patients to support the production of red blood cells and manage anemia.

4. Phosphate Binders

- **Calcium-based binders (e.g., Calcium Carbonate):** These medications bind to phosphate in the digestive tract and prevent its absorption, helping to control high phosphate levels that can lead to bone disorders in kidney disease patients.

- **Non-calcium-based binders (e.g., Sevelamer):** These are used to avoid excess calcium intake, especially in patients who are at risk of vascular calcification.

5. Potassium Binders

- **Sodium Polystyrene Sulfonate (e.g., Kayexalate):** This medication is used in cases where potassium levels become dangerously high, which is a risk in later stages of kidney disease.

Over-the-Counter (OTC) Medications & Their Impacts

Over-the-counter (OTC) medications are widely used for a variety of common ailments, such as pain, colds, and headaches. However, for individuals with stage 3 kidney disease, certain OTC medications can pose significant risks to kidney health. It's crucial for seniors and caregivers to understand which medications are safe and which should be avoided or used with caution.

1. Nonsteroidal Anti-Inflammatory Drugs (NSAIDs)

Examples: Ibuprofen (Advil, Motrin), Naproxen (Aleve)

- **Impact:** NSAIDs are commonly used for pain relief and reducing inflammation. However, they can reduce blood flow to the kidneys, potentially causing acute kidney injury, especially in cases where kidney function is already compromised. They can also lead to increased blood pressure and fluid retention, which exacerbates kidney disease.

- **Alternative:** Acetaminophen (Tylenol) is generally considered safer for pain relief in kidney disease patients, as it has less impact on kidney function. However, it should be used cautiously and within recommended dosage limits to avoid liver damage.

2. Antacids and Laxatives

Examples: Magnesium-based antacids (Milk of Magnesia), Sodium Phosphate Enemas

- **Impact:** Some antacids and laxatives contain magnesium or phosphate, which can accumulate in the body if kidney function is impaired, leading to serious health issues such as hypermagnesemia or hyperphosphatemia.

- **Alternative:** For antacids, H2 blockers like ranitidine or proton pump inhibitors like omeprazole may be safer alternatives but should still be used under medical advice. For laxatives, those containing polyethylene glycol are usually safer options.

3. Cold and Flu Medications

Examples: Multi-symptom cold and flu products

- **Impact:** Many OTC cold and flu medications contain a mix of ingredients, including decongestants such as pseudoephedrine, which can increase blood pressure, and NSAIDs. These components can pose risks for individuals with kidney disease.

- **Alternative:** Choosing single-ingredient medications appropriate for specific symptoms is advised. For example, using a nasal saline spray instead of a decongestant for congestion can be a safer choice.

4. Herbal Supplements and Nutritional Supplements

- **Impact:** While not traditional OTC medications, many individuals take supplements that are available over the counter. Supplements such as herbal diuretics, potassium, and certain vitamins can alter kidney function or interact negatively with kidney medications.

It's essential to consult with a doctor before starting any new supplement, especially if you have kidney disease, to ensure it won't interfere with kidney function or other medications.

Herbal Supplements and Kidney Health

The use of herbal supplements is popular for their perceived benefits and natural origins. However, for individuals with stage 3 kidney disease, it's essential to approach herbal supplements with caution, as some can have harmful effects on kidney function or interact with medications. Here, we'll explore common herbal supplements, their potential risks, and safer alternatives.

1. High-Risk Herbal Supplements

- **Licorice Root:** While often used for digestive issues and sore throats, it can be harmful to people with kidney disease. Licorice root can raise blood pressure and decrease potassium levels, which can be dangerous for those with kidney problems.

- **Astragalus:** This herb is used to boost the immune system, but it can act as a diuretic (increasing urine production), potentially dehydrating the body. It can also interact with medications that affect the immune system and blood pressure.

- **St. John's Wort:** Commonly used for depression, St. John's Wort can interfere with the metabolism of many medications, including immunosuppressants taken by transplant patients. This interaction can reduce the effectiveness of the medication or lead to potentially harmful side effects.

2. **Moderately Risky Herbal Supplements**

- **Turmeric:** Turmeric, a vibrant yellow spice, is often touted for its anti-inflammatory properties, and some research suggests it might benefit kidney health. However, turmeric contains oxalates, which can contribute to kidney stone formation in susceptible individuals. While using turmeric as a spice in cooking is generally safe, it's important to be cautious with high-dose turmeric supplements, especially if you have a history of kidney stones or other kidney issues. It's best to discuss the use of turmeric supplements with your doctor or renal dietitian, as they can advise you on a safe dosage or alternative options that might be better suited to your needs.

- **Ginger:** Ginger is a versatile spice known for its anti-inflammatory and digestive benefits. However, in larger doses (often found in supplements or concentrated extracts), it may act as a mild blood thinner and interact with medications like warfarin. It's generally safe to use ginger in typical culinary amounts, like adding it to dishes or beverages. However, if you're taking blood thinners or have concerns about your kidney health, it's crucial to talk to your doctor about using ginger supplements or consuming large amounts of ginger. You will be guided on safe usage and potential interactions with your medications.

3. **Safer Herbal Alternatives**

- **Cranberry:** Cranberry, whether enjoyed as a juice, supplement, or dried fruit, is often associated with urinary tract health due to its potential to prevent bacteria from adhering to the urinary tract lining. Some studies suggest it may even offer kidney health benefits due to its antioxidant and anti-inflammatory properties. However, it's important to remember that cranberry is not a treatment for existing urinary tract infections. If you suspect a UTI, reach out to your doctor for diagnosis and treatment. Also, excessive consumption of cranberry, particularly in the form of juice, can increase the risk of kidney stones in some individuals. Moderation and choosing unsweetened options are key for those with Stage 3 CKD.

- **Chamomile:** Chamomile tea is known for its soothing properties and is often used for relaxation and sleep promotion. It's generally considered safe for those with kidney disease, but it can have a mild blood-thinning effect. This means it might not be suitable if you're taking blood thinners like warfarin. If you enjoy chamomile tea and are on any medications, it's crucial to discuss it with your doctor to ensure it won't interfere with your treatment plan.

Medications to Avoid or Use With Caution

If you have Stage 3 kidney disease, it's important to be extra careful with certain medications, as they can sometimes put extra strain on your kidneys. Here are a few types to be particularly mindful of:

1. **Pain Relievers (NSAIDs):** Common over-the-counter pain relievers like ibuprofen (Advil, Motrin) and naproxen (Aleve) can sometimes decrease blood flow to the kidneys. This can be risky if your kidney function is already reduced. If you need pain relief, talk to your doctor about safer alternatives or non-medication options like heat therapy or gentle exercise.

2. **Certain Antibiotics:** Some antibiotics, especially those called aminoglycosides and certain sulfonamides, need to be used cautiously as they can potentially harm your kidneys. Your doctor will choose the safest antibiotic for you and adjust the dosage if necessary.

3. **Contrast Dye (for Imaging Tests):** The dye used in some tests like CT scans and MRIs can sometimes affect kidney function, especially if you already have kidney disease. Talk

to your doctor about any upcoming tests and whether some alternative options or precautions can be taken.

4. **Laxatives (Especially in Large Amounts):** Taking laxatives too often or in high doses can lead to dehydration and upset the balance of minerals in your body. This can strain your kidneys. If you experience constipation, talk to your doctor about gentle, kidney-friendly options and lifestyle changes that can help.

5. **Potassium-Sparing Diuretics:** These "water pills" can be helpful for reducing swelling and lowering blood pressure, but they can also increase potassium levels. If you're taking this type of diuretic, your doctor will monitor your bloodwork closely and help you make any necessary adjustments to your diet or medications.

6. **Supplements with Potassium or Magnesium:** Even some over-the-counter supplements can contain high amounts of potassium or magnesium. Since your kidneys might have a harder time removing these minerals, too much can build up in your blood. Always check with your doctor before starting any new supplement, and be sure to read the labels carefully.

This isn't a complete list, but it covers some common medications to be cautious about. The most important thing is to be an active participant in your healthcare. Talk to your doctor and pharmacist about all the medicines you're taking, ask questions, and let them know about any side effects you experience.

CHAPTER 13

LIFESTYLE CHANGES FOR OPTIMAL KIDNEY HEALTH

Managing Stage 3 kidney disease isn't just about what's on your plate. A healthy lifestyle plays a crucial role in supporting your kidneys, boosting your overall well-being, and improving your quality of life. This chapter will explore key lifestyle factors that work hand-in-hand with your diet to keep you feeling your best. We'll discuss practical ways to manage stress, monitor your health, get a good night's sleep, and build a strong support network. Remember, small changes can make a big difference, and you're not alone in this journey!

Practical Stress Management Strategies for Seniors

Stress is a natural part of life, but when you're managing Stage 3 kidney disease, it can feel particularly overwhelming. It's important to understand how stress can affect your kidneys and overall health, and to find effective ways to manage it.

How Stress Impacts Your Kidneys

Stress triggers the release of hormones like cortisol and adrenaline, which are designed to help your body respond to threats. However, when stress becomes chronic or overwhelming, these hormones can wreak havoc on your health, including your kidneys.

- **Increased Blood Pressure:** Stress hormones can cause your blood vessels to constrict, leading to a spike in blood pressure. Over time, high blood pressure can damage the delicate blood vessels in your kidneys, making it harder for them to filter waste and perform their essential functions.

- **Reduced Kidney Blood Flow:** Stress can also decrease blood flow to your kidneys, depriving them of oxygen and nutrients needed for optimal function.

- **Worsening Existing Conditions:** If you have other health conditions like diabetes or high blood pressure, stress can exacerbate them, further impacting your kidney health.

- **Weakened Immune System:** Chronic stress can suppress your immune system, making you more susceptible to infections and other illnesses.

- **Sleep Problems:** Stress can lead to difficulty falling asleep or staying asleep, contributing to fatigue and decreased energy levels.

- **Poor Appetite & Digestion:** Stress can disrupt your appetite and digestive processes, making it harder to get the nutrients your body needs.

- **Increased Inflammation:** Stress is linked to inflammation throughout the body, including in the kidneys. This can contribute to tissue damage and worsen kidney function.

- **Mental Health Concerns:** Chronic stress can exacerbate anxiety and depression, creating a vicious cycle where emotional distress further impacts physical health.

Relaxation Techniques for Seniors

The good news is that you have the power to manage stress and protect your kidneys! Here are some simple yet effective techniques specifically tailored for seniors:

Deep Breathing Exercises: Deep breathing can help calm your mind and body. Take a comfortable seat, close your eyes, and inhale deeply through your nose for a count of four. Hold the same breath for the same four counts; gradually release it through your mouth for another four counts. Continue doing this repeatedly until you start to feel more relaxed.

Mindfulness Meditation: Mindfulness involves focusing on the present moment and accepting it without judgment. It can help reduce stress and improve your mental well-being. You can start by sitting quietly and focusing on your breath. If your mind strays, gently return your focus to your breathing. There are many apps, like Headspace or Calm, that offer guided mindfulness sessions to help you get started.

Progressive Muscle Relaxation: This system involves tensing and then gently releasing each muscle group in your body. Start with your toes and work your way up to your head. This technique can aid in promoting relaxation and easing bodily stress.

Yoga and Tai Chi: These gentle physical activities combine movement, breath control, and meditation. They can help improve flexibility, reduce stress, and enhance your overall well-being. Many community centers and gyms offer classes tailored for beginners or seniors.

Walking in Nature: Spending time outdoors in nature can be very calming. Even a short walk in a park or garden can help you feel more relaxed and connected to the world around you.

Key Health Indicators for Healthier Kidneys

Staying on top of your health is key when managing Stage 3 kidney disease. By keeping a close eye on certain key indicators, you can work hand-in-hand with your healthcare team to make informed decisions and adjust your treatment plan if needed. Here's what to watch out for:

Your Blood Pressure

Your blood pressure is a measure of how hard your heart works to pump blood throughout your body. When it's high, it puts extra strain on your kidneys and can worsen kidney disease. That's why it's important to know your numbers and check your blood pressure regularly – either at home or at the doctor's office, depending on what your doctor recommends.

Keep track of your readings in a simple log or journal, noting any patterns or changes. This helps you and your doctor see how things are going over time. If your numbers are consistently high, or if you experience symptoms like dizziness or headaches, be sure to talk to your doctor. Managing your blood pressure is a team effort, and they're there to help you make the right adjustments to your lifestyle and medications if needed.

Healthy Weight Balance

Maintaining a healthy weight is crucial for your overall health and is especially important when managing kidney disease. Extra weight puts additional strain on your kidneys, so aiming for a healthy range can make a big difference.

Talk to your doctor or dietitian to determine what weight is right for you. Then, make a habit of weighing yourself regularly and keeping track of the numbers. Remember, a balanced, kidney-friendly diet and regular physical activity are the keys to achieving and maintaining a healthy weight.

If you're finding it challenging to manage your weight, don't hesitate to reach out to your healthcare team. They can provide support, guidance, and resources to help you reach your goals!

Other Key Indicators to Monitor

- **Blood Sugar:** If you have diabetes, managing your blood sugar levels is crucial for protecting your kidneys. Monitor your blood sugar regularly as recommended by your doctor.

- **Fluid Balance:** If your doctor has recommended fluid restrictions, keep track of your intake to prevent fluid buildup.

- **Kidney Function Tests:** Your doctor will likely recommend regular blood and urine tests to monitor how well your kidneys are functioning. These tests help assess the effectiveness of your treatment plan and make necessary adjustments.

- **Medication Side Effects:** Pay attention to any side effects you experience while taking your medications and discuss them with your doctor.

Healthy Sleep Hygiene for Healthy Kidneys

Sleep is more than just a time for rest. It's a crucial part of staying healthy, especially when managing kidney disease. Quality sleep allows your body to repair and recharge, supporting your immune system, energy levels, and even your kidney function. Here are some tips to help improve your sleep hygiene:

1. **Create a Routine**: Consistency is key to good sleep. Make an effort to go to bed and get up at the same time daily, even on weekends. This helps regulate your body's internal clock and can improve the quality of your sleep.

2. **Create a Sleep-friendly Environment**: Your bedroom should be a haven for rest. Keep it dark, quiet, and cool. If need be, shut off any distractions with blackout curtains, a white noise machine, or earplugs.

3. **Reduce Screen Time Before Bed**: The blue light from computers, phones, and tablets can make it hard for you to sleep. Be intentional about keeping away from screens an hour before bedtime. Instead, engage in a relaxing activity, such as reading a book or listening to soothing music.

4. **Avoid Stimulants**: Restrict your caffeine and nicotine intake, particularly in the afternoon and evening. These substances can disrupt your sleep. Instead, opt for a calming herbal tea, like chamomile, in the evening.

5. **Relax Before Bed**: Develop a pre-sleep routine that helps you unwind. This could include taking a warm bath, practicing gentle yoga, or doing some light stretching. Engaging in these activities can help signal to your body that it's time to relax and get ready for bed.

The Power of Building Social Support Network

When facing the challenges of Stage 3 kidney disease, having a strong support system can make a world of difference. Connecting with others who understand your journey can offer comfort, encouragement, and valuable information. Here's how to build and maintain a supportive network:

1. **Join Support Groups**: Connecting with others who are going through similar experiences can be incredibly helpful. Look for local or online support groups for people with kidney disease. These groups provide a safe space to share your

feelings, exchange tips, and gain insights from others who understand what you're going through.

2. **Communicate with Loved Ones**: Share your experiences and challenges with family and friends. Educate them about your condition so they can offer appropriate support. Let them know how they can help you, whether it's accompanying you to doctor's appointments, helping with meal preparation, or simply being there to listen.

3. **Engage in Social Activities**: Stay involved in community activities and hobbies you enjoy. This can improve your mood, provide a sense of normalcy, and help you stay connected with others. Whether it's joining a book club, listening to music, participating in a walking group, or volunteering, find activities that bring you joy and fulfillment.

4. **Seek Professional Help**: If you feel overwhelmed, consider talking to a counselor or therapist who specializes in chronic illness. They can help you manage your emotions, develop coping strategies, and provide a safe space to express your feelings.

Changing your lifestyle helps you to control your health and provide the greatest possible support for your kidneys. Remember that every good decision you make, whether big or small, adds up to improve your quality of life.

CHAPTER 14

EXERCISE & PHYSICAL ACTIVITY FOR KIDNEY HEALTH

One of the most crucial things you can do for your general health—especially if you have stage 3 chronic kidney disease (CKD)—is to keep active. Exercise enhances your mental health, energy level, quality of life, and physical well-being. For seniors, regular physical activity is essential for maintaining independence, managing symptoms, and enjoying a higher quality of life. This chapter will explore the many benefits of exercise, recommend safe and effective types of exercises, and provide tips to keep you charged and motivated to make exercise a regular part of your routine.

The Value of Exercises to Seniors with Stage 3 CKD

Engaging in regular physical activity offers numerous benefits that are especially important for seniors with stage 3 CKD. Here's how exercise can positively impact your health:

1. **Improves Cardiovascular Health**: Regular exercise strengthens the heart and improves circulation, and thus helps to manage high blood pressure—a common issue for those with CKD. Lower blood pressure reduces the strain on your kidneys and can slow the progression of kidney disease.

2. **Enhances Muscle Strength and Flexibility**: Maintaining muscle strength and flexibility is crucial for daily activities and preventing falls. Exercise helps keep your muscles and joints strong and flexible, and this helps to promote better mobility and reduces the risk of injuries.

3. **Aids Weight Management**: Exercise helps burn calories and maintain a healthy weight. Being overweight can exacerbate CKD and other health conditions like diabetes and hypertension. Regular exercise can help you achieve and maintain a healthy weight, reducing stress on your kidneys.

4. **Improves Mental Health**: Physical activity releases endorphins, which are natural mood lifters. Exercise can reduce symptoms of depression and anxiety, boost your mood, and improve your overall mental well-being. It can also provide a sense of accomplishment and purpose.

5. **Enhances Sleep Quality**: Regular physical activity can help regulate your sleep patterns, making it easier to fall asleep and stay asleep. Better sleep contributes to overall health and well-being, including kidney health.

6. **Boosts Energy Levels**: Exercise improves your endurance and overall energy levels, making it easier to perform daily tasks and engage in activities you enjoy.

Safe & Effective Exercises to Enjoy

It's essential to choose exercises that are safe, enjoyable, and suitable for your fitness level. Find below some types of activities that are particularly considered beneficial for seniors with stage 3 CKD:

1. **Walking**: Walking is a low-impact exercise that is easy to do and doesn't require special equipment. It's a great way to improve cardiovascular health, strengthen muscles, and boost your mood. Start with short walks and progressively increase the time and intensity as your fitness improves.

2. **Swimming and Water Aerobics**: Water-based exercises are gentle on the joints and can provide a full-body workout. Swimming and water aerobics can help improve cardiovascular fitness, muscle strength, and flexibility without putting too much strain on your body.

3. **Tai Chi and Yoga**: These gentle, low-impact activities focus on balance, flexibility, and breathing. They can help reduce stress, improve balance, and increase strength and flexibility. Many classes are tailored specifically for seniors, making them a great option.

4. **Strength Training**: Light strength training exercises can help maintain and build muscle mass, which is important for overall health and mobility. Use light weights or resistance bands, and focus on exercises that work for all major muscle

groups. Always start with low resistance and gradually increase as you become stronger.

5. **Cycling**: Using a stationary bike or a regular bicycle can be an excellent cardiovascular workout that's easy on the joints. It is a great way to improve your heart health and leg strength.

6. **Chair Exercises**: For those with limited mobility, chair exercises can provide a safe and effective way to stay active. These exercises can help improve strength, flexibility, and circulation while minimizing the risk of falls.

Tips for Making Exercise a Habit

It might be difficult to incorporate exercise into your routine on a daily basis, but with the right techniques, it can become a fun and enduring habit. Here are some pointers to keep you motivated:

1. **Set Realistic Goals**: Begin with small, attainable goals and progressively increase your activity level. Setting realistic goals helps build confidence and keeps you motivated as you see progress.

2. **Find Activities You Enjoy**: Choose exercises that you find enjoyable and fun. You're more likely to stick with activities that you look forward to rather than those you see as a chore.

3. **Make it Social**: Exercising with friends, family, or in a group can make physical activity more enjoyable and provide a sense of accountability. Join a walking group, attend a fitness class, or find a workout buddy to stay motivated.

4. **Create a Routine**: Schedule your exercise sessions at the same time each day to build a routine. Consistency is key to forming a long-term habit.

5. **Track Your Progress**: Keeping a record of your activities and progress can help you stay motivated and see how far you've come. Use a journal, an app, or a fitness tracker to log your workouts.

6. **Reward Yourself**: Celebrate your achievements with non-food rewards. When you hit your fitness targets, treat yourself to something special, like a soothing bath or a fun outing.

7. **Listen to Your Body**: Pay attention to how your body feels during and after exercise. It's important to exercise at a pace that feels comfortable and safe for you. If you experience pain or discomfort, modify your activity or take a break.

8. **Seek Professional Guidance**: Consider working with a physical therapist or a fitness trainer who has experience

with seniors and chronic conditions. They can help you create a personalized exercise plan that's safe and effective.

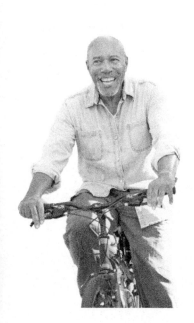
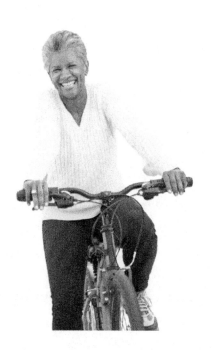

21-DAY EXERCISE PLAN

This 21-day exercise plan is designed specifically for seniors with stage 3 CKD. It provides a balanced mix of walking, strength training, and flexibility exercises, all tailored to be safe, effective, and enjoyable. Each day's activities are carefully planned to ensure they are manageable, avoiding any overwhelming routines while promoting consistent physical activity.

By following this plan, you'll gradually build a habit of regular exercise that will help to improve your kidney health and overall well-being. Remember to listen to your body, stay hydrated, and enjoy the journey towards a healthier, more active lifestyle.

Remember to always consult your doctor before starting any new exercise routine.

Week 1

Day 1: Walking

- 15-20 minutes of walking at a comfortable pace
- Stretching: 5 minutes of gentle stretching focusing on legs and back

Day 2: Rest Day

- Light activity such as leisurely walking or household chores

Day 3: Strength Training

- Seated leg lifts: 1 set of 10 reps
- Bicep curls with light weights: 1 set of 10 reps

- Wall push-ups: 1 set of 10 reps
- Stretching: 5 minutes

Day 4: Rest Day

- Light activity such as leisurely walking or household chores

Day 5: Walking

- 15-20 minutes of walking at a comfortable pace
- Stretching: 5 minutes

Day 6: Flexibility and Balance

- Gentle yoga or Tai Chi: 15-20 minutes
- Stretching: 5 minutes

Day 7: Rest Day

- Light activity such as leisurely walking or household chores

Week 2

Day 8: Walking

- 20-25 minutes of walking at a comfortable pace
- Stretching: 5 minutes

Day 9: Rest Day

- Light activity such as leisurely walking or household chores

Day 10: Strength Training

- Seated marches: 1 set of 10 reps
- Shoulder presses with light weights: 1 set of 10 reps
- Heel raises: 1 set of 10 reps

- Stretching: 5 minutes

Day 11: Rest Day

- Light activity such as leisurely walking or household chores

Day 12: Walking

- 20-25 minutes of walking at a comfortable pace
- Stretching: 5 minutes

Day 13: Flexibility and Balance

- Chair yoga: 15-20 minutes
- Stretching: 5 minutes

Day 14: Rest Day

- Light activity such as leisurely walking or household chores

Week 3

Day 15: Walking

- 25-30 minutes of walking at a comfortable pace
- Stretching: 5 minutes

Day 16: Rest Day

- Light activity such as leisurely walking or household chores

Day 17: Strength Training

- Seated leg lifts: 1 set of 12 reps
- Bicep curls with light weights: 1 set of 12 reps
- Wall push-ups: 1 set of 12 reps
- Stretching: 5 minutes

Day 18: Rest Day

- Light activity such as leisurely walking or household chores

Day 19: Walking

- 25-30 minutes of walking at a comfortable pace
- Stretching: 5 minutes

Day 20: Flexibility and Balance

- Gentle yoga or Tai Chi: 15-20 minutes
- Stretching: 5 minutes

Day 21: Rest Day

- Light activity such as leisurely walking or household chores

Tips for Success

1. **Listen to Your Body**: Adjust the intensity and duration of exercises based on how you feel. Avoid overexertion.

2. **Stay Hydrated**: Drink plenty of water before, during, and after exercise.

3. **Warm-Up and Cool Down**: Always start with a warm-up and end with a cool down to prevent injuries and muscle soreness.

4. **Consistency**: Aim to follow the plan consistently, but don't be discouraged if you miss a day. Just pick up where you left off.

Seek Support: If possible, exercise with a friend or join a group to stay motivated and make the experience more enjoyable.

30 DAYS MEAL PLAN

Day 1:

- **Breakfast:** Apple Cinnamon Oatmeal **(p. 48)**
- **Lunch:** Turkey and Cheese Wrap **(p. 60)**
- **Dinner:** Lemon Herb Grilled Salmon **(p. 78)**
- **Snack:** Zucchini Sticks **(p. 94)**

Day 2:

- **Breakfast:** Cottage Cheese with Pineapple **(p. 50)**
- **Lunch:** Apple Cranberry Walnut Salad **(p. 62)**
- **Dinner:** Cauliflower Rice Stir-Fry **(p. 80)**
- **Snack:** Apple Cinnamon Chips **(p. 95)**

Day 3:

- **Breakfast:** Baked Apple Oatmeal **(p. 51)**
- **Lunch:** Balsamic Marinated Mushrooms **(p. 61)**
- **Dinner:** Quinoa Stuffed Bell Peppers **(p. 81)**
- **Snack:** Pear & Almond Parfait **(p. 105)**

Day 4:

- **Breakfast:** Vegetable Omelet **(p. 49)**
- **Lunch:** Baked Salmon with Dill **(p. 63)**

- **Dinner:** Minestrone Soup (p. 87)

- **Snack:** Crispy Kale Chips (p. 98)

Day 5:

- **Breakfast:** Zucchini Bread (p. 52)

- **Lunch:** Roasted Asparagus & Wild Mushroom Stew (p. 64)

- **Dinner:** Baked Tilapia with Fresh Herbs (p. 88)

- **Snack:** Flour Tortilla Chips (p. 101)

Day 6:

- **Breakfast:** Quinoa Breakfast Bowl (p. 53)

- **Lunch:** Vegetable Stir-Fry with Tofu (p. 65)

- **Dinner:** Pork Tenderloin with Apple Chutney (p. 89)

- **Snack:** Baked Apple Wedges (p. 99)

Day 7:

- **Breakfast:** Peach Compote Toast (p. 54)

- **Lunch:** Pasta Primavera (p. 66)

- **Dinner:** Roasted Chicken with Herbs (p. 91)

- **Snack:** Carrot and Celery Sticks (p. 102)

Day 8:

- **Breakfast:** Easy Chia Seed Pudding (p. 55)

- **Lunch:** Mediterranean Quinoa Salad with Roasted Summer Vegetables **(p. 70)**

- **Dinner:** Tropical Chicken Risotto **(p. 79)**

- **Snack:** Coleslaw **(p. 100)**

Day 9:

- **Breakfast:** Bulgur Wheat Porridge **(p. 56)**

- **Lunch:** Chicken Tortilla Casserole **(p. 72)**

- **Dinner:** Broccoli with Garlic and Lemon **(p. 85)**

- **Snack:** Pineapple Bar Cookies **(p. 102)**

Day 10:

- **Breakfast:** Spicy Tofu Scrambler **(p. 56)**

- **Lunch:** Mushroom Barley Soup **(p. 71)**

- **Dinner:** Lentil Soup with Spinach **(p. 90)**

- **Snack:** Granola Bars **(p. 103)**

Day 11:

- **Breakfast:** Avocado Toast **(p. 58)**

- **Lunch:** Zucchini Tortilla Bites **(p. 73)**

- **Dinner:** Cobb Salad **(p. 92)**

- **Snack:** Low-Sodium Flour Tortilla Chips **(p. 104)**

Day 12:

- **Breakfast:** Cherry Almond Chia Pudding **(p. 57)**

- **Lunch:** Baked Turkey Spring Rolls **(p. 68)**

- **Dinner:** Cranberry Pecan Rice Pilaf **(p. 82)**

- **Snack:** Baked Tofu Cubes **(p. 107)**

Day 13:

- **Breakfast:** Low-Sodium Pancakes **(p. 59)**

- **Lunch:** Tropical Chicken Risotto **(p. 74)**

- **Dinner:** Mushroom and Spinach Risotto **(p. 86)**

- **Snack:** Pear & Almond Parfait **(p. 105)**

Day 14:

- **Breakfast:** Creamy Rice Pudding **(p. 48)**

- **Lunch:** Chipotle Shrimp Tacos **(p. 76)**

- **Dinner:** Chinese-Style Asparagus **(p. 84)**

- **Snack:** Roasted Cauliflower and Green Bean Bites **(p. 97)**

Day 15:

- **Breakfast:** Vegetable Frittata **(p. 53)**

- **Lunch:** Vegetable Stir-Fry with Tofu **(p. 65)**

- **Dinner:** Baked Tilapia with Fresh Herbs **(p. 88)**

- **Snack:** Apple Caramel Crisp **(p. 106)**

Day 16:

- **Breakfast:** Apple Cinnamon Oatmeal **(p. 48)**

- **Lunch:** Pasta Primavera **(p. 66)**

- **Dinner:** Pork Tenderloin with Apple Chutney **(p. 89)**

- **Snack:** Pineapple Bar Cookies **(p. 102)**

Day 17:

- **Breakfast:** Zucchini Bread **(p. 52)**

- **Lunch:** Balsamic Marinated Mushrooms **(p. 61)**

- **Dinner:** Roasted Chicken with Herbs **(p. 91)**

- **Snack:** Cucumber Sandwiches **(p. 95)**

Day 18:

- **Breakfast:** Quinoa Breakfast Bowl **(p. 53)**

- **Lunch:** Mushroom Barley Soup **(p. 71)**

- **Dinner:** Quinoa Stuffed Bell Peppers **(p. 81)**

- **Snack:** Carrot and Celery Sticks **(p. 102)**

Day 19:

- **Breakfast:** Peach Compote Toast **(p. 54)**

- **Lunch:** Turkey and Cheese Wrap **(p. 60)**

- **Dinner:** Lentil Soup with Spinach **(p. 90)**

- **Snack:** Flour Tortilla Chips **(p. 101)**

Day 20:

- **Breakfast:** Easy Chia Seed Pudding **(p. 55)**
- **Lunch:** Mediterranean Quinoa Salad with Roasted Summer Vegetables **(p. 70)**
- **Dinner:** Cauliflower Rice Stir-Fry **(p. 80)**
- **Snack:** Baked Apple Wedges **(p. 99)**

Day 21:

- **Breakfast:** Bulgur Wheat Porridge **(p. 56)**
- **Lunch:** Chicken Tortilla Casserole **(p. 72)**
- **Dinner:** Cranberry Pecan Rice Pilaf **(p. 82)**
- **Snack:** Crispy Kale Chips **(p. 98)**

Day 22:

- **Breakfast:** Spicy Tofu Scrambler **(p. 56)**
- **Lunch:** Apple Cranberry Walnut Salad **(p. 62)**
- **Dinner:** Broccoli with Garlic and Lemon **(p. 85)**
- **Snack:** Granola Bars **(p. 103)**

Day 23:

- **Breakfast:** Avocado Toast **(p. 58)**
- **Lunch:** Roasted Asparagus & Wild Mushroom Stew **(p. 64)**
- **Dinner:** Tropical Chicken Risotto **(p. 79)**

- **Snack:** Zucchini Sticks (p. 94)

Day 24:

- **Breakfast:** Cherry Almond Chia Pudding (p. 57)

- **Lunch:** Vegetable Stir-Fry with Tofu (p. 65)

- **Dinner:** Minestrone Soup (p. 87)

- **Snack:** Low-Sodium Flour Tortilla Chips (p. 104)

Day 25:

- **Breakfast:** Low-Sodium Pancakes (p. 59)

- **Lunch:** Baked Turkey Spring Rolls (p. 68)

- **Dinner:** Baked Tilapia with Fresh Herbs (p. 88)

- **Snack:** Apple Caramel Crisp (p. 106)

Day 26:

- **Breakfast:** Creamy Rice Pudding (p. 48)

- **Lunch:** Chipotle Shrimp Tacos (p. 76)

- **Dinner:** Pork Tenderloin with Apple Chutney (p. 89)

- **Snack:** Roasted Cauliflower and Green Bean Bites (p. 97)

Day 27:

- **Breakfast:** Vegetable Frittata (p. 53)

- **Lunch:** Turkey and Cheese Wrap (p. 60)

- **Dinner:** Roasted Chicken with Herbs (p. 91)

- **Snack:** Coleslaw (p. 100)

Day 28:

- **Breakfast:** Apple Cinnamon Oatmeal (p. 48)
- **Lunch:** Mediterranean Quinoa Salad with Roasted Summer Vegetables (p. 70)
- **Dinner:** Mushroom and Spinach Risotto (p. 86)
- **Snack:** Cucumber Sandwiches (p. 95)

Day 29:

- **Breakfast:** Zucchini Bread (p. 52)
- **Lunch:** Apple Cranberry Walnut Salad (p. 62)
- **Dinner:** Lentil Soup with Spinach (p. 90)
- **Snack:** Flour Tortilla Chips (p. 101)

Day 30:

- **Breakfast:** Quinoa Breakfast Bowl (p. 53)
- **Lunch:** Chicken Tortilla Casserole (p. 72)
- **Dinner:** Cauliflower Rice Stir-Fry (p. 80)
- **Snack:** Baked Tofu Cubes (p. 107)

MEASUREMENT AND CONVERSIONS

Volume Equivalents (Dry)

US STANDARD	METRIC (APPROX.)
⅛ teaspoon	0.5 mL
¼ teaspoon	1 mL
½ teaspoon	2 mL
¾ teaspoon	4 mL
1 teaspoon	5 mL
1 tablespoon	15 mL
¼ cup	59 mL
⅓ cup	79 mL
½ cup	118 mL
⅔ cup	156 mL
¾ cup	177 mL
1 cup	235 mL
2 cups or 1 pint	475 mL
3 cups	700 mL
4 cups or 1 quart	1 L
½ gallon	2 L
1 gallon	4 L

Volume Equivalents (Liquid)

US STANDARD	US STANDARD (OUNCES)	METRIC (APPROX)
2 tablespoons	1 fl. oz.	30 mL
¼ cup	2 fl. oz.	60 mL
½ cup	4 fl. oz.	120 mL
1 cup	8 fl. oz.	240 mL
1½ cups	12 fl. oz.	355 mL
2 cups or 1 pint	16 fl. oz.	475 mL
4 cups or 1 quart	32 fl. oz.	1 L
1 gallon	128 fl. oz.	4 L
16 fl. oz. 475 mL	16 fl. oz. 475 mL	16 fl. oz.

OVEN TEMPERATURES

FAHRENHEIT (F)	CELSIUS (C) (APPROX.)
250°F	120°C
300°F	150°C
325°F	165°C
350°F	180°C
375°F	190°C
400°F	200°C
425°F	220°C
450°F	230°C

WEIGHT EQUIVALENTS

US STANDARD	METRIC (APPROX)
½ ounce	15 g
1 ounce	30 g
2 ounces	60 g
4 ounces	115 g
8 ounces	225 g
12 ounces	340 g
16 ounces or 1 pound	455 g

CONCLUSION

Well, here we are at the end of this cookbook, but really, it's just the start of your journey toward a healthier, more vibrant life with Stage 3 kidney disease.

Remember when you first picked up this book? Think about how much you've learned since then. You're practically a pro at understanding your kidneys, the impact of your diet, and making food choices that truly support you. Give yourself a big pat on the back—you've made incredible progress!

But let's be honest: managing kidney disease isn't something that happens overnight. It's a marathon, not a sprint. There will be days that are smooth sailing and others that might be a bit tougher. The trick is to be kind to yourself, celebrate every little win, and always reach out for support when you need it. Your healthcare team, your family, your friends—they're all cheering you on.

And this cookbook? It's more than just a bunch of recipes. It's your trusty partner in the kitchen, your ticket to exploring a world of flavors and possibilities. Keep diving into those recipes, experiment with new ingredients, and find joy in making meals that nourish both your body and soul.

Food isn't just about filling your belly. It's about pleasure, connection, and celebrating life. By embracing a kidney-friendly diet, you're not giving anything up—instead, you're adding more joy to your days and more life to your years.

This is just the beginning of your journey. With the knowledge you've gained, the support you have, and a positive attitude, you're more than capable of thriving with Stage 3 kidney disease.

And if you ever have questions or just want to share how your cooking adventures are going, don't hesitate to reach out. You'll find my email at the top of the book.

Here's to delicious meals, good health, and a life filled with joy!

THANK YOU

Thank you once again for choosing the **Kidney Disease Diet for Seniors on stage 3** as your guide on this journey.

If you found this book helpful, I would greatly appreciate it if you could leave a positive review. Your review will help others who are looking for a guide to manage their chronic kidney disease.

Thank you again for your support.

ACCESS TO MY OTHER BOOKS

I have other books that you could find helpful. Kindly scan the code below to gain access.

OR https://www.amazon.com/author/michgreen

BONUS

WEEKLY MEAL PLANNER

Weekly Meal Planner

Date: _____

	BREAKFAST	LUNCH	DINNER	SNACKS
MON				
TUE				
WED				
THU				
FRI				
SAT				
SUN				

SHOPPING LIST

- _____
- _____
- _____
- _____
- _____
- _____
- _____

NOTES

○
○
○
○
○

Weekly Meal Planner

Date: _____

	BREAKFAST	LUNCH	DINNER	SNACKS
MON				
TUE				
WED				
THU				
FRI				
SAT				
SUN				

SHOPPING LIST

- _____
- _____
- _____
- _____
- _____
- _____
- _____
- _____

NOTES

Weekly Meal Planner

Date: _____

	BREAKFAST	LUNCH	DINNER	SNACKS
MON				
TUE				
WED				
THU				
FRI				
SAT				
SUN				

SHOPPING LIST

- _____
- _____
- _____
- _____
- _____
- _____
- _____
- _____

NOTES

○
○
○
○
○

Weekly Meal Planner

Date: _____

	BREAKFAST	LUNCH	DINNER	SNACKS
MON				
TUE				
WED				
THU				
FRI				
SAT				
SUN				

SHOPPING LIST

- _____
- _____
- _____
- _____
- _____
- _____
- _____
- _____

NOTES

○
○
○
○
○
○

Weekly Meal Planner

Date: _____

	BREAKFAST	LUNCH	DINNER	SNACKS
MON				
TUE				
WED				
THU				
FRI				
SAT				
SUN				

SHOPPING LIST

- _____
- _____
- _____
- _____
- _____
- _____
- _____
- _____

NOTES

○
○
○
○
○

Weekly Meal Planner

Date: _____

	BREAKFAST	LUNCH	DINNER	SNACKS
MON				
TUE				
WED				
THU				
FRI				
SAT				
SUN				

SHOPPING LIST

- _____
- _____
- _____
- _____
- _____
- _____
- _____
- _____

NOTES

Weekly Meal Planner

Date: _____

	BREAKFAST	LUNCH	DINNER	SNACKS
MON				
TUE				
WED				
THU				
FRI				
SAT				
SUN				

SHOPPING LIST

- _____
- _____
- _____
- _____
- _____
- _____
- _____
- _____

NOTES

Weekly Meal Planner

Date: _____

	BREAKFAST	LUNCH	DINNER	SNACKS
MON				
TUE				
WED				
THU				
FRI				
SAT				
SUN				

SHOPPING LIST

- _____
- _____
- _____
- _____
- _____
- _____
- _____
- _____

NOTES

○
○
○
○
○
○

Weekly Meal Planner

Date: _____

	BREAKFAST	LUNCH	DINNER	SNACKS
MON				
TUE				
WED				
THU				
FRI				
SAT				
SUN				

SHOPPING LIST

- _____
- _____
- _____
- _____
- _____
- _____
- _____
- _____

NOTES

○ _____
○ _____
○ _____
○ _____
○ _____
○ _____

Weekly Meal Planner

Date: _____

	BREAKFAST	LUNCH	DINNER	SNACKS
MON				
TUE				
WED				
THU				
FRI				
SAT				
SUN				

SHOPPING LIST

- _____
- _____
- _____
- _____
- _____
- _____
- _____
- _____

NOTES

- ○
- ○
- ○
- ○
- ○

Printed in Great Britain
by Amazon